Physical Examination of the Newborn
at a Glance

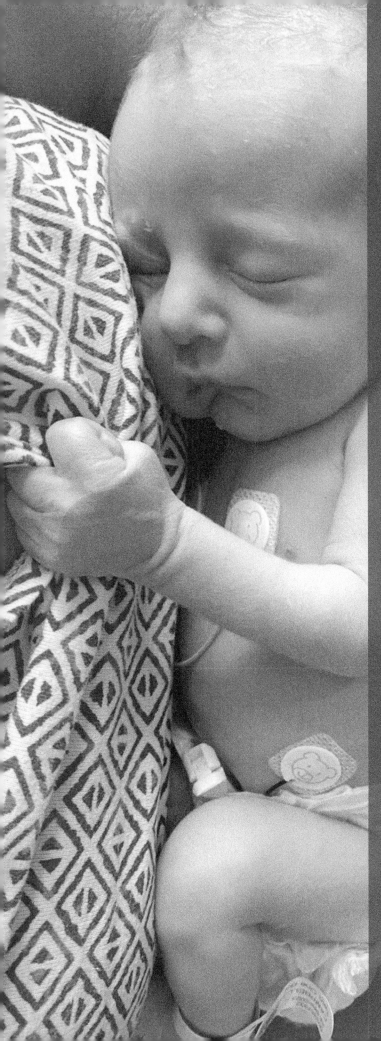

Physical Examination of the Newborn

at a Glance

Second Edition

Dr Lyn Dolby EdD
RN, RM, MSc, FHEA
Senior Lecturer and Course Leader
in Midwifery
Anglia Ruskin University
Northampton, UK

Denise (Dee) Campbell
RN, RM, BSc, PgDip, MA, FHEA
Principal Lecturer and Programme Tutor in
Midwifery (*retired*)
Hertfordshire University
Hatfield, UK

Series Editor
Ian Peate OBE, FRCN

WILEY Blackwell

Contents

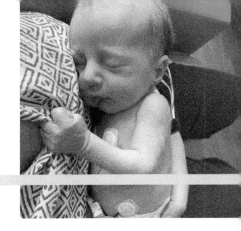

Part 6 Revision and self-assessment   125

Section 15 Revision activities: crosswords and
multiple-choice questions

Section 16 Self-assessment: professional reflection

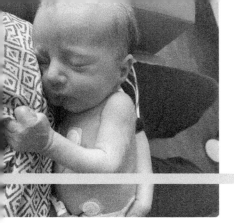

Preface

This is the second edition of *Physical Examination of the Newborn at a Glance*. Both healthcare students and qualified staff find it useful to have a resource that they can dip into as part of their initial learning or to serve as an update. This new edition has been updated and expanded as the result of feedback from the first edition and the contemporary information that is now available. As a result, this edition includes new chapters relating to health promotion from a professional point of view, and neonatal adaptation has been split into two: information for parents and extra information for students and practitioners. There are new chapters covering 'Professionalism and leadership' and 'Genetics and inheritance'. Useful insights into some of the misconceptions that exist in professional midwifery practice have also been highlighted within the text.

At times this new edition will hopefully make you, the reader, think about what professionalism is, the language we as professionals use and when we need to change our perceptions and conversations because of new knowledge and insight. To this end, some original chapters have been replaced by two chapters instead of one due to the quantity of research that is now available in order to aid in clarity.

In relation to the newborn baby and in particular the newborn and infant physical examination (PHE, 2021a), the role of effective communication and good working relationships with paediatricians are paramount if the baby is to be referred and treated in a timely manner and the parent(s) are to feel satisfied that they are being adequately informed and supported. Some Trust sites demonstrate very effective and respectful working relationships, whereas others are unfortunately not renowned for such collegiate working. Therefore, aspects of professionalism and leadership have been introduced in this edition to provoke thought in relation to what your profession and professionalism mean – in other words, why do you work as you do, do you feel that you can practise according to the standard of the knowledge and skill that you have achieved or does the environmental culture (behaviour and communication) create barriers to effective practice?

Reflection 'on' and 'in' practice is an important and expected part of professional practice. Therefore, as professionals you need to review whether your NHS Trust service provision is 'fit for purpose' in relation to the needs of your clients and what continuity of care should 'look like' for the clients who access the maternity and obstetric services in your area. In some areas of the United Kingdom, NIPE midwives can experience frustration in relation to referral processes and so on, whereas in other NHS Trust sites this is not the case, which begs the question of why. In addition, there is recognition of the need to raise the equity of the experience, standard and quality of care to both parents and their babies (NHS England, 2023c).

It is important that you acknowledge the extent of your professional knowledge within the workplace and that other disciplines respect the standard you have achieved in much the same manner as you should respect theirs. After all, leadership does not mean that you have to be a manager. Essentially a leader is a professional who recognises an issue and starts a discussion with others about how the situation can be improved or resolved. As a professional, not doing anything is not a choice, as it would mean that you have chosen to become part of the problem instead of part of the solution.

Ultimately, both of us hope that this second edition not only assists you in raising your level of knowledge, but also makes you think about your autonomous role and that raising your leadership activities (NMC, 2018), whether in relation to students or colleagues, is just as important!

Abbreviations

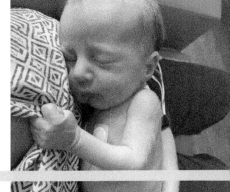

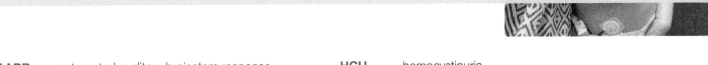

AABR	automated auditory brainstem response
ACTH	congenital adrenal hyperplasia
ADH	anti-diuretic hormone
AFP	alpha-fetoprotein
AHT	abusive head trauma
ANNB	Antenatal and Newborn
AOAE	automated otoacoustic emissions
BAPM	British Association of Perinatal Medicine
BAT	brown adipose tissue
BCG	bacille Calmette–Guérin
BMI	body mass index
BN	Bohn's nodules
BP	blood pressure
CF	cystic fibrosis
cfDNA	cell-free DNA
CHD	congenital heart defect
CHT	congenital hypothyroidism
CMV	cytomegalovirus
CNS	central nervous system
CONI	Care of the Next Infant
CSC	children's social care
CSF	cerebro-spinal fluid
CVS	chorionic villus sampling
DAT	direct antiglobulin test
DDH	developmental dysplasia of the hips
DHSC	Department of Health and Social Care
DIC	disseminated intravascular coagulation
DNA	deoxyribonucleic acid
ECTG	electronic cardiotocography
EEG	electroencephalogram
elfh	elearning for healthcare
EP	Epstein pearls
FAS	fetal alcohol syndrome
FASP	fetal anomaly screening programme
FISH	fluorescent in-situ hybridisation
G6PD	glucose-6-phosphate dehydrogenase deficiency
GA1	glutaric aciduria type 1
GBS	group B *Streptococcus*
GMC	General Medical Council
GP	general practitioner
HAI	healthcare-acquired infection
HCU	homocystinuria
HDN	haemolytic disease of the newborn
HIV	human immunodeficiency virus
HR	heart rate
HSV	herpes simplex virus
HV	health visitor
ICON	Infant crying is normal, Comforting methods can help, it is OK to walk away, Never, ever shake a baby
IMD	inherited metabolic disease
IO	intra-osseous
IRT	infrared thermography
IT	information technology
IUGR	intrauterine growth retardation
IV	intravenous
IVA	isovaleric acidaemia
KPI	key performance indicator
LSP	Local Safeguarding Partner
MCADD	medium-chain acyl-coenzyme A dehydrogenese deficiency
MORA	Midwifery Ongoing Record of Achievement
MSUD	maple syrup urine disease
MW	midwife
NBCP	National Bereavement Care Pathway
NBS	newborn blood spot
NEWTT2	Newborn Early Warning Trigger and Track
NHS	National Health Service
NICE	National Institute for Health and Care Excellence
NICU	neonatal intensive care unit
NIPE	newborn and infant physical examination
NMC	Nursing and Midwifery Council
NQM	newly qualified midwife
NSC	National Screening Committee
OAV	oculo-auricular-vertebral
PCHR	personal child health record
PCR	polymerase chain reaction
PGE2	prostaglandin
PHE	Public Health England
PKU	*phenylketonuria*
PMA	Professional Midwifery Advocate
PPHN	persistent pulmonary hypertension of the newborn

PROM	premature rupture of membranes		**SEN**	systematic examination of the newborn
PVP	programmable ventriculo-peritoneal		**SIDS**	sudden infant death syndrome
RBC	red blood cell		**SUDI**	sudden unexpected death in infancy
S4N	SMaRT4NIPE		**TB**	tuberculosis
SBC	spina bifida cystica		**TcB**	transcutaneous bilirubinometer
SBO	spina bifida occulta		**TSB**	total serum bilirubin
SBR	serum bilirubin		**TSH**	thyroid-stimulating hormone
SCBU	special care baby unit		**USS**	ultrasound scan
SCD	sickle cell disease		**VZV**	varicella zoster virus
SCID	severe combined immunodeficiency			

Professional issues

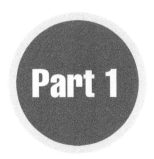

Part 1

Chapters

Public health screening and the neonate

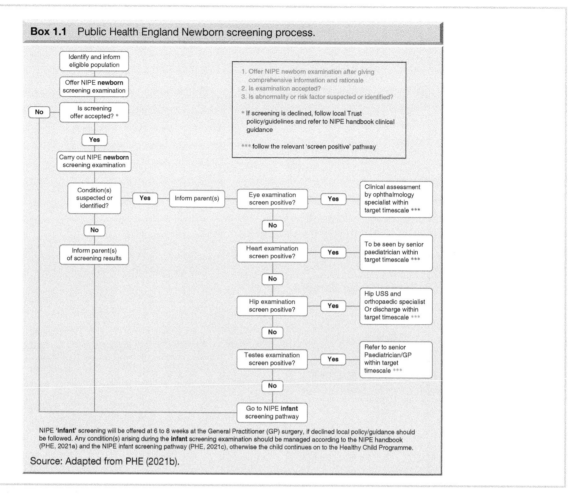

Box 1.1 Public Health England Newborn screening process.

Identify and inform eligible population

Offer NIPE **newborn** screening examination

Is screening offer accepted? * — No

Yes

Carry out NIPE **newborn** screening examination

Condition(s) suspected or identified? — Yes → Inform parent(s)

No

Inform parent(s) of screening results

1. Offer NIPE newborn examination after giving comprehensive information and rationale
2. Is examination accepted?
3. Is abnormality or risk factor suspected or identified?

* If screening is declined, follow local Trust policy/guidelines and refer to NIPE handbook clinical guidance

*** follow the relevant 'screen positive' pathway

Eye examination screen positive? — Yes → Clinical assessment by ophthalmology specialist within target timescale ***

No

Heart examination screen positive? — Yes → To be seen by senior paediatrician within target timescale ***

No

Hip examination screen positive? — Yes → Hip USS and orthopaedic specialist Or discharge within target timescale ***

No

Testes examination screen positive? — Yes → Refer to senior Paediatrician/GP within target timescale ***

No

Go to NIPE **infant** screening pathway

NIPE '**infant**' screening will be offered at 6 to 8 weeks at the General Practitioner (GP) surgery, if declined local policy/guidance should be followed. Any condition(s) arising during the **infant** screening examination should be managed according to the NIPE handbook (PHE, 2021a) and the NIPE infant screening pathway (PHE, 2021c), otherwise the child continues on to the Healthy Child Programme.

Source: Adapted from PHE (2021b).

The UK National Screening Committee (NSC) advises ministers and the National Health Service (NHS) in the four UK countries in relation to all aspects of screening. It supports implementation, updating and standards across a range of screening programmes in an ethical and evidence-based manner. The NSC reviews the patient experience of the screening process and their journey to referral (PHE, 2022).

The newborn and infant physical examination (NIPE) is one of the programmes within its remit. This term clearly denotes that screening for newborn health (Box 1.1) relates to the **newborn** examination (carried out by 72 hours of life) and the **infant** examination (usually conducted within the general practice [GP] surgery from 6 to 8 weeks of life). The term NIPE is also used on NSC-related documentation, including guidance and referral pathways. However, it is worth noting that where the national Midwifery Ongoing Record of Achievement (MORA) is used for student midwife training, it is referred to as the systematic examination of the newborn (see Chapter 4 for further clarification). Also, the term NIPE is not consistently used in Scotland but is used in some other countries internationally, although it should be remembered that the content and expectation of the examination may not be the same as those guided

by the NIPE handbook (PHE, 2021a). Therefore, when employing international midwives it is important to ascertain what they were taught and the content and standard of the course they have undertaken in comparison to UK standards prior to active practice.

The NSC draws evidence from world-class research and by promoting advocacy and collaborative partnerships, all of which assist in the delivery of specialist public health services. It also has close liaison with the Screening Quality Assurance Service, which audits the achievement of national standards and verifies that screening programmes remain safe and effective. Furthermore, NHS Trusts and NIPE practitioners can inform their knowledge and support best practice by accessing the *Newborn and infant physical examination (NIPE) screening programme handbook* (PHE, 2021a) and the *Newborn and infant physical examination (NIPE) newborn screening pathway* (PHE, 2021b). *Both* of these texts are updated and amended to reflect the available evidence and therefore it is important that practitioners refer to the latest edition. It is also important that the guidance document, *Newborn and infant physical examination screening pathway requirements specification* (Office for Health Improvement and Disparities, 2021), is referred to in the same manner.

Physical Examination of the Newborn at a Glance, Second Edition. Dr Lyn Dolby and Denise (Dee) Campbell.
© 2025 John Wiley & Sons Ltd. Published 2025 by John Wiley & Sons Ltd.

Screening not diagnosis

Population screening provides access to a process of identifying healthy people who may be at increased risk of a disease or condition. In the event that an individual may be highlighted as being at a higher risk of developing the disease or condition, they can then receive further information, investigations and/or treatment. The provision of screening aims to reduce the risks or complications associated with a disease or condition.

Screening is *not* a diagnostic process. Without further investigation, a screening process cannot usually provide confirmation that an individual has a specific disease or condition. However, newborn blood spot screening is an exception as screening is offered for all babies, thus there will be some babies in whom a specific condition is confirmed and where treatment and management of the condition will be offered.

In relation to NIPE, there are four main screening elements that are assessed: eyes, heart, hips and testes. This is not because examining the baby for other conditions is not important, but rather because these four elements can be systematically measured and therefore standards relating to good practice and time scales can be set accordingly. However, this does not mean that the opportunity to assess the baby's overall condition (e.g. skin, abdomen, reflexes etc.) is unimportant and the same care and attention should be exercised in relation to the overall examination and the findings recorded. The Personal Child Health Record reflects this requirement, as space is allocated to enable this process and provide a record for parents, community midwives, health visitors and the family GP.

Programme requirements

NHS Trusts are required to have processes in place whereby all eligible babies are offered the NIPE within 72 hours of birth. A second 'infant' physical examination is offered again at 6 to 8 weeks of age by the family's GP (PHE, 2021c). However, it is the responsibility of the provider in whose area the baby was born to identify all eligible babies (including those who move into the area) in order to offer the 72-hour NIPE and identify whether it has been completed, or whether responsibility for it has been transferred to another acute care provider. The responsibility for following up on referrals after the 6-week examination rests with the GP, who should check the care pathway for progression in relation to referrals or results of action taken.

The main aim of the NIPE programme is to detect congenital abnormalities of the eyes, heart, hips and testes, where these are detectable within the first 72 hours after birth. The examination at 6 to 8 weeks provides a second opportunity to detect these abnormalities and it also occurs at the time when the neonatal period ends. The ending of the neonatal period is in alignment with the completion of most of the physiological changes that occur after birth. Most babies will have completed the transition from fetal to neonatal life and therefore conditions arising after this time will not necessarily be congenital in origin, plus some conditions may not present with any signs or symptoms at the time of the earlier examination for the practitioner to act on. However, if an abnormality is undetected or masked by another condition or illness, then it may still be first recognised due to parental concern or because the baby exhibits signs and symptoms of its presence. It is a salient point to note that parental concerns should be taken seriously – they know their child and changes in behaviour or ability will often be clear to them.

Parental information

All parents should be given information relating to the NIPE in terms of what it is, why it is offered, when it is performed and by whom. During the antenatal period and before the NIPE is conducted, a leaflet should be provided and discussion should take place so that questions can be answered and to give the parents time to think about any family history of which the practitioner may not yet be aware. Parents also need to be know who has access to the information documented in relation to the examination, to enable them to make their decision about whether to consent to the examination or not in an informed manner. There is **no reason**, in relation to NIPE, that parents should not be given the necessary information together with time for questions and to discuss their thoughts with others prior to consenting for the examination to take place. Asking for permission (consent) is part of professional practice, demonstrates respect for individual wishes and beliefs and alludes to the requirements of the law of the country in which the examination is taking place. Consent should be noted within all documentation and on the SMaRT4NIPE (S4N) system (if available in the area). S4N provides an information and audit trail that also highlights actions that may be required in relation to findings recorded, as well as babies born who have not been recorded as having their NIPE completed by the signposted time periods.

During the examination, the ability of their baby should be mentioned and any concerns that the parents may have should be addressed. The findings of the examination should be discussed with the parents prior to the practitioner completing a comprehensive record (see Chapter 3 on documentation). They should also be made aware of who they can contact if they have concerns about their baby's health and that the second screening examination will be when the baby is 6 to 8 weeks of age, when any further questions should be asked. For example, the baby may have had unilateral undescended testis at the 72-hour examination and the parents will need to know if this has now resolved, or they may have a concern that has arisen since the newborn examination that needs to be addressed.

Key considerations

NIPE guidance (PHE, 2021a) recommends that the 72-hour examination should be undertaken on all babies prior to their discharge home. This maximises the likelihood that the examination will be completed in a timely manner. It is also advantageous for the parents, as some will not want to return to the hospital after having gone home. There will also be some who will choose not to return and not to take part in screening now that they are no longer in the environment where it is most usually offered.

If an examination must be performed early in neonatal life when auscultating heart murmurs is more likely, it is preferential to do so rather than the examination not be conducted. As with a baby at any point in the first 72 hours and beyond this time parameter, there is always the possibility of hearing a heart murmur and therefore the information given in relation to signs of ill health is no less or more important for one baby during this time than any other. Thus, there is no reason that the examination cannot be performed soon after birth if the parents wish to go home.

If a baby has been admitted to a neonatal intensive care unit (NICU) or special care baby unit (SCBU), then all practitioners who come into contact with the baby should ensure that the neonate does not miss out on the examination and that the rationale for any delay is comprehensively documented. If a baby has been discharged home from the NICU/SCBU, then the practitioners in the community such as the midwife, health visitor or GP need to investigate whether the NIPE has been comprehensively completed, as sometimes it can be missed.

As with any programme, the completion of all its components is paramount and the S4N system will assist in highlighting errors or omissions. However, the process of completion will still only be as good as the attention to detail of the professionals involved.

2 Quality, standards, thresholds and audit

Table 2.1 Standards and performance thresholds relating to the newborn physical examination.

Standard	Descriptor	Performance thresholds
NIPE-S01: coverage	The proportion of babies eligible who are tested (where offer is accepted) for all four NIPE components (three in female infants) at ≤72 hours of age and have a conclusive result on day of report	Acceptable level: ≥95.0% Achievable level: ≥97.5%
NIPE-S02: Diagnosis/intervention – timeliness of intervention for babies with screen-positive results	The proportion of babies with a screen-positive eye result who attend clinical assessment by an ophthalmology specialist within ≤2 weeks of the examination	Acceptable level: ≥95.0% Achievable level: ≥99.0%
NIPE-S03: Diagnosis/intervention – timeliness of ultrasound scan of the hips for developmental dysplasia	The proportion of babies with a screen-positive newborn hip result who attend for ultrasound scan of the hips within the designated time scale[b]	Acceptable level: ≥90.0% Achievable level: ≥95.0%
NIPE-S04: Diagnosis/intervention – timeliness of hip clinical assessment or discharge	The proportion of babies with a screen-positive newborn hip result at newborn physical examination for whom an outcome decision was made within the designated time scale[a] N.B. Excludes those babies who die prior to USS or who are found to have 'clicky hip'	None set at present
NIPE-S05: Diagnosis/intervention – timeliness of intervention for bilateral undescended testes	The proportion of babies: Identified with bilateral undescended testes detected at newborn physical examination Seen by a consultant paediatrician or associate specialist within ≤24 hours post newborn examination	Acceptable level: 100%

[a] Caveats are in place for these standards relating to gestational age at birth – see *NIPE programme handbook* (PHE, 2021a).
Source: Adapted from OHID (2021).

Table 2.2 Audit requirements in relation to Trust site pathway outcome.

Providers must have systems in place to:

- Use the NIPE national IT system to record all screening and follow-up data
- Regularly check that all screening results are recorded on the NIPE national IT system (referred to as SMaRT4NIPE or S4N) in line with national guidance
- Identify and follow up all babies who have not competed the NIPE screening pathway (see Section 7: Babies who have missed screening in the *Newborn and infant physical examination (NIPE) screening programme handbook* (PHE, 2021a)
- Review local screening outcome and data quality reports to enable surveillance and audit of data quality and completeness
- Provide data and reports mapped against programme standards, key performance indicators and quality indicators as required, to monitor all outcomes

NHS Trusts utilise a systematic approach to maintain and improve the quality of patient care while reducing risk. To achieve these aims, robust processes are put in place to facilitate the audit of areas such as clinical effectiveness, education and training, risk management and transparency in relation to investigation and policy. In effect, quality assurance provides a process that enables continuous audit of progress, standard of practice and/or activity and the identification of issues that require improvement. Quality assurance assists in assessing whether the standards set are not only being met but are also appropriate and feasible.

Each of the NHS national screening programmes has its own clearly defined set of standards. However, in order that the process of quality assurance is robust and comprehensive, several factors should be considered. First, a screening programme is developed and overseen by a committee of people who have experience and knowledge in that specific field of expertise or who have first-hand knowledge (professionals and service users). Facilitating a quality review of the service includes diverse participants such as those involved in commissioning or providing screening services as well as those who use the service.

The committee assists in the development of national quality standards. This involves setting up processes that can monitor how the service meets (or not) the standards set. In the event of adverse incidents, the committee also provides access to expert screening advice to allow for effective incident management.

Quality assurance is all-encompassing and covers the screening process from start to finish. This process commences with the premise that the screening programme is justifiable; it decides who will be offered screening; it continues throughout the screening activity and, if required, referral for further investigation. In relation to the NIPE, the main aim is to provide a screening service that is accessible to all parents and their babies and for a minimum standard to be maintained in order to minimise harm while maximising the benefit derived from screening.

A consistent driver within quality assurance is the need to maintain a high-quality service. Collaboration with local screening programmes through the involvement of local teams is important. Effective team working necessitates that professionals, commissioners and the screening committee work towards risk reduction and ensure that audit trails are working effectively. A process that works well should be able to respond appropriately to incidents, allow productive inter-professional communication to take place if the issue is to be resolved and promote the sharing of good practices.

Quality assurance is inevitably a formal process and each local screening programme is responsible for its own effectiveness.

This is monitored by statistical review, regional meetings or even informal visits. The NIPE standards give a parameter to work towards, which is feasible and allows for the very slight local differences that occur from region to region. However, it should be noted that NIPE **infant** screening (PHE, 2021c) is not formally managed and has no national standards for this particular examination, as systematic measurement is difficult to accomplish. Therefore, local commissioners oversee and provide scrutiny as required.

Audit processes

Key performance indicators (KPIs) were introduced into NHS screening programmes to assist in the measurement of performance within specific areas. They act as a tool to govern and assess performance by helping to identify potential or actual problems. Highlighting issues is important if the root cause is to be uncovered and a solution found to remedy the situation. Table 2.1 provides an overview of the main standards and the performance thresholds that are deemed 'acceptable' and 'achievable' (OHID, 2021). Therefore, if the thresholds are not being met, the Trust site is obliged to investigate and resolve the issue in a timely and appropriate manner that is sustainable. For example, it is possible that there are too few experienced NIPE practitioners available to help support those who are newer to the role, or it could be that data is missing. In the former instance, reassessing the training or updating available for staff or providing 'buddies' for newly trained staff can resolve the issue. However, in the latter instance it could be that at times it is difficult for staff to access the NIPE national information technology (IT) system (known as SMaRT4NIPE or S4N). Therefore an adequate back-up process needs to be in place that is clearly signposted for all staff, so that adequate documentation of the NIPE examination findings can be transferred to S4N when the system eventually comes back online and so that the parents are adequately informed of actions taken. At other times, further advice will need to be accessed if more specific or unique issues arise.

The use of S4N enables data to be collected that identifies areas of shortfall, near misses or those areas where clinical performance is exemplary. Table 2.2 indicates how audit is applied to pathway outcomes for those Trust sites using S4N, but those Trust sites where S4N is not yet operational have had to put in place their own methods for auditing the standards. Practitioners should refer to the specification pathways requirements specification (OHID, 2021) that outlines the areas of data collection for audit requirements, as these areas may also be used for research.

3 Documentation

Figure 3.1 The personal child health record.

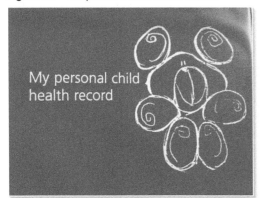

My personal child health record

Figure 3.2 Pages within the personal child health record relating to the newborn examination.
Source: CROWN COPYRIGHT / https://www.blmkhealthiertogether.nhs.uk/application/files/6616/1356/1037/167711_v4.5_PCHR_FINAL_complete_Dec_19.pdf, last accessed 11 May 2024/ CC BY 3.0.

Birth details & newborn examination – page 1 of 3

* Please place a sticker (if available) otherwise write in space provided.

Surname:
First names:
NHS number: Unit no:
Address: Sex: M / F
                Post code: D.O.B: ...../...../
G.P: Code:
H.V: Code:

Place of birth:
Length of pregnancy in weeks:
Type of delivery:
Mother's NHS Number:
Problems in pregnancy, birth or neonatal period:
Admitted to Neonatal Intensive Care Unit? ☐

Birth Weight: ....kg Length: ....cm *(if indicated)* Head circumference: ....cm Date: ...../...../
Consent: Consent given ☐ Declined ☐

Newborn Examination

Item	Guide to Content	Results		Action Taken	
Examination of hips	Barlow & Ortolani tests on both Check for DDH	Condition suspected If yes:	Yes ☐ No ☐ Left ☐ Right ☐	Referred	Yes ☐ No ☐
Examination of eyes	Includes inspection and red reflex	Condition suspected If yes:	Yes ☐ No ☐ Left ☐ Right ☐	Referred	Yes ☐ No ☐
Examination of heart	Includes colour, pulses, heart sounds, murmurs etc.	Condition suspected Pulse Oximetry performed	Yes ☐ No ☐ Yes ☐ No ☐	Referred	Yes ☐ No ☐
Testes	Look for undescended testes	Condition suspected If yes:	Yes ☐ No ☐ Left ☐ Right ☐	Referred	Yes ☐ No ☐

Risk factors present Yes ☐ No ☐   Risk factor details *(if family history, state relative)*..............

Date Performed: .... Performed by: .... Signature: ....

Top copy: remain in PCHR   2nd Copy: Health Visitor   3rd Copy: Child Health Department

Birth details and newborn examination – page 1 of 3

3

Birth details & newborn examination – page 2 of 3

* Please place a sticker (if available) otherwise write in space provided.

Surname:
First names:
NHS number: Unit no:
Address: Sex: M / F
                Post code: D.O.B: ...../...../
G.P: Code:
H.V: Code:

First milk feed:
Breast ☐   Formula ☐

Breastfeeding at discharge:
Totally ☐ Partially ☐ Not at all ☐

Date of discharge: ...../...../

Newborn examination (contd)

Item	Guide to Content	Results	Action taken
Rest of physical examination	Includes: fontanelle, palate, spine, abdomen, urine system, passage of meconium etc.	Condition suspected Yes ☐ No ☐ If yes, details:	Referred Yes ☐ No ☐ If yes, details:

Newborn Bloodspot Screening Programme

Date blood taken ...../...../   (results and further details on page 31-32)

Top copy: remain in PCHR   2nd Copy: Health Visitor   3rd Copy: Child Health Department

Birth details and newborn examination – page 2 of 3

3a

Physical Examination of the Newborn at a Glance, Second Edition. Dr Lyn Dolby and Denise (Dee) Campbell.
© 2025 John Wiley & Sons Ltd. Published 2025 by John Wiley & Sons Ltd.

Every practitioner is responsible for the records that they make, the care and information that they give, the rationale for actions they take and the summarised discussions that occur both between parent(s) and practitioners and between healthcare professionals. When completing the appropriate records on the examination of the newborn, the same diligence and attention to detail apply to this part of one's professional role (NMC, 2018) as to the rest of one's professional practice. Whether the examination relates to the initial examination of the newborn, the daily newborn examination or the NIPE, all relevant documentation must be completed.

The findings of the examination and a summary of the salient points of discussion between the parents and the practitioner, including any parental concerns and the reassurance or information given at the time, should be clearly documented. Parents must always be informed, if relevant, as to who will have access to their child's record, which can include midwives, paediatricians, health visitors and social workers.

Both the Nursing and Midwifery Council (NMC, 2018) and the General Medical Council (GMC, 2012) provide guidance on professional and ethical practice, which incorporates the principles of effective documentation and communication. These principles include the following key elements:

• Documentation should be clear, comprehensive and easily understandable.
• All entries to records must be signed by the person who gave practical care or information. In the case of written records, most Trust site records (including the National Neonatal Notes) provide a section to complete with the name of the practitioner (in block capitals), their designation and signature to enable easy identification. Digital records have an automatic digital record of who entered the record and/or made an entry. In the case of SMaRT4NIPE (S4N) documentation, the practitioner who conducted the NIPE must check that the name identified is correct.
• The date and time should be given for every recorded entry and this should be in real time and in chronological order. The entry should be made as contemporaneously as possible, being as close to the actual time as would be considered feasible in the eyes of the law. For example, it should not take three hours to record the findings of an examination unless, for example, an emergency occurred or S4N was inaccessible, in which case the reason for the delay should be documented in the notes.
• Records must be accurate and recorded in such a way that the meaning is clear, factual and must not include unnecessary or non-standard abbreviations, jargon, meaningless phrases or irrelevant speculation.

• Records should provide an accurate summary of activity, findings, discussion and information given to parent(s) and other healthcare professionals, management plans and actions taken.
• The parent(s) should be aware of the findings that the practitioner is recording within the notes and the practitioner must assess if they understand what is said and what it means. Parents need to have access to comprehensive information for the wellbeing of both them and their baby. If the parent(s)' first language is not English, then use of an interpreting service is paramount.
• If a written record is being used, entries should be chronological and legible and written in black ink pen, in case there is a need for the record to be photocopied or scanned. Any alterations, additions or changes to the plan of care should be clearly marked as such, with accompanying date, time and rationale.

Documentation relating to NIPE

In general, the documents that are completed in relation to the NIPE include the local NHS Trust Neonatal Notes and digital record, the personal child health record (PCHR) and the S4N system, which was set up by the NSC to assist in the capture of data relating to the NIPE for audit and failsafe purposes. More information on the failsafe standards can be obtained via the local NHS Trust Antenatal and Newborn (ANNB) failsafe officer.

The PCHR is given to the parents for each child (Figures 3.1 and 3.2 highlight the relevant sections). It is a document that is frequently updated in line with current practice and today's technology. The contemporary version can be accessed via the website listed with Figure 3.2. It should also be noted that even with the available digital technology, the paper version of the PCHR is still available in order to allow all parents equal access.

It should be noted that the S4N system is external to the NHS Trust. Therefore, it is paramount that a back-up system enabling the NIPE practitioner to complete a paper record is easily accessible if the system itself is inaccessible (PHE, 2021h). This can occur due to S4N system failure or because the system is being updated. Parents must be informed that the PCHR has been completed and a separate paper record of the findings has been made, that a note has been placed on the Trust Neonatal Notes and that the digital document will be completed as soon as the system is back online. Both staff in the relevant areas and the screening nurse need to know about the event, as they will need to ensure that the information is posted on the S4N system at the earliest opportunity, while ensuring that the name of the NIPE practitioner who conducted the examination is correct on the entry. An effective process will ensure that it will not be assumed that a baby has missed the newborn examination.

4 Professionalism and leadership

Figure 4.1 What do these words mean to you in your professional role?

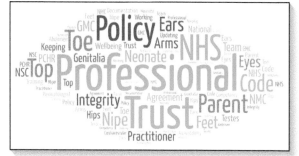

Box 4.1 Useful websites for professional knowledge.

Newborn and infant physical examination (NIPE) screening programme handbook (updated 2021)
https://www.gov.uk/government/publications/newborn-and-infant-physical-examination-programme-handbook/newborn-and-infant-physical-examination-screening-programme-handbook

Newborn and infant physical examination (NIPE) newborn screening pathway (updated 2021)
https://www.gov.uk/government/publications/newborn-and-infant-physical-examination-programme-handbook/newborn-and-infant-physical-examination-nipe-infant-screening-pathway

Newborn and infant physical examination: training requirements. Guidance for NHS providers of maternity and neonatal services on training requirements regarding newborn and infant physical examination (NIPE) (2023)
https://www.england.nhs.uk/long-read/newborn-and-infant-physical-examination-training-requirements

NMC – The Code (2018)
https://www.nmc.org.uk/globalassets/sitedocuments/nmc-publications/nmc-code.pdf

Box 4.2 Professional issues that cause frustration in relation to the newborn and infant physical examination (NIPE) – where do you and your NHS Trust stand?

- Midwifery and paediatric policies are not linked or, at times, one discipline can only access their own
- Criteria on which babies midwives are 'allowed' to conduct NIPEs vary. Some Trust sites exclude all but term baby born spontaneously per vaginum and booked caesarean section births, whereas at the other end of the spectrum others have wider criteria that only exclude babies with obvious health issues or abnormality
- On some Trust sites a midwife can refer a baby for hip risk factors (no positive signs on examination) for ultrasound scan (USS), but on others the referral will not be accepted in ultrasonography without a doctor's signature. Is this appropriate or should the doctor complete their own investigation and examination prior to completing a USS referral?
- Do junior doctors receive theoretical training and adequate, supervised practical time, or is it a 'see one and do one' approach? How do you feel about the quality of supervision for junior doctors in relation to your own NIPE course?
- Who completes the information on the Personal Child Health Record?
- Are all practitioners expected to complete the NIPE online learning via the elearning for healthcare (elfh) hub? Are NIPE update sessions easily accessible?
- Do all practitioners investigate the records for family, obstetric and neonatal history prior to the examination?

Examination of the newborn comes in many forms, such as the initial newborn examination, the daily examination, as well as those examinations that sit under the umbrella of the NIPE – the newborn examination (by 72 hours of age) and the infant examination (by 6 to 8 weeks of age). All of these need a professional explanation and agreement of the parents before the examination takes place. The professional role and responsibility of the practitioner and student need to be as respected as the legal implications attached to them. However, the NIPE must only be completed by a healthcare professional who has been appropriately trained to provide the duty of care and skill required. The healthcare professionals who can conduct the NIPE include members of the paediatric team, advanced neonatal nurse practitioners, GPs, midwives and student midwives working under supervision with a NIPE practitioner (in those areas where a complete course in NIPE is part of their programme of learning). Although far more universities already include training for NIPE within their foundation pre-registration programmes of midwifery, others will be expected to do so as their courses are updated in the future.

Figure 4.1 uses some of the key words associated with the varying healthcare disciplines. As reflection should be an essential part of any professional practice, this is a good point to think about which words epitomise most strongly what your professional role means to you and those for whom you have a professional responsibility and accountability for their well-being. You may see certain words, such as referral or team, in a positive light within your workplace, or conversely they may make a negative impact on your ability to work in a professional manner. Importantly, you need to be able to see what works in your workplace and what needs to be resolved, what misconceptions are apparent about the roles of different disciplines and whether the workforce is prepared to be proactive in the process of change.

Newborn and infant physical examination or systematic examination of the newborn?

The national Midwifery Ongoing Record of Achievement (MORA) is currently used by many but not all universities that provide a foundation midwifery programme. This document does align to the NMC Standards for Proficiency of Midwives (NMC, 2019), but only provides a record of completion in relation to the 'systematic physical examination of the newborn' (SEN) and therefore there needs to be a clear understanding that this does not confirm that the individual has completed theory and practice in NIPE. In an attempt to clarify the situation, NHS England (2023a) issued a statement in relation to training requirements, but unfortunately there are some NMC practitioners within universities who perceive that SEN within the MORA constitutes a confirmed record of practical training achievement for NIPE, as though this is an updated term. Also the term NIPE is not universal, for example Scotland developed the Scottish Routine Examination of the Newborn course and in some countries the term NIPE is used but may not reflect the same expectations as in the United Kingdom, for example skills in relation to practical assessment of the cardiovascular system may not be taught within the training. Therefore, it is paramount that the NMC, NSC, Trust sites and university staff pay attention to the confusion that can occur due to terminology. It is also important that practitioners are aware what the terms NIPE and SEN actually represent, thus it is worth reading the NHS England (2023a) publication relating to training requirements (see Box 4.1 regarding useful websites to access for further information).

Professionalism and leadership

There is another issue of growing concern that the NSC may not fully appreciate in relation to the need for there to be a stronger emphasis on the supervision of junior doctors, particularly regarding the hip assessment, health promotion and documentation. Midwives are often very vocal in relation to the perceived competence of junior doctors, especially when referring a baby to a senior paediatrician who sends a junior doctor instead. They often feel that this shows little respect for the level of theoretical and practical knowledge they have achieved when completing their NIPE, although they appreciate that there are not enough senior paediatric staff (Dolby, 2023). Unfortunately, this aspect does have an impact on how midwifery staff view medical staff attitudes towards them and on interprofessional communication, which has been a factor in inhibiting some midwives from continuing to conduct NIPEs. Therefore, there is a clear need to support midwives in practice in order to improve relationships between paediatricians and midwives while developing resilient midwives in the present and in the future. This is paramount if both students and midwives are to see themselves as autonomous professionals in their own right and as leaders of change rather than bystanders. Admittedly, midwives have stated that they are aware that a change needs to occur and that they require managerial and executive Trust support to do this, if they are to work as they feel they have been trained to do (Dolby, 2023).

Proactive leadership is not the sole domain of managers; it is in the hands of a collective professional body. Managers need to listen to midwives and midwives need to clearly state their requirements to managers and then work together to resolve issues in practice. For example, the provision of opportunities for all NIPE and student practitioners (no matter their discipline) to get together to discuss issues as a team has worked well and proved productive in changing negative workplace cultures, which in turn has provided students with a sense of what interdisciplinary collaboration and communication should be like (Dolby, 2023). However, it is recognised that this requires facilitators of change to have innovative and effective leadership skills if they are to foster an environment that promotes and encourages collaborative working that continues to be supported and encouraged in everyday practice. Therefore, change has to occur in protocols and the behaviour of medical, midwifery and ultrasonography staff and at Trust executive level. There also needs to be a national discussion about the criteria concerning the babies on which midwives can complete NIPEs (Box 4.2), as there is a disparity across Trust sites, even with those that are only a few miles apart.

Trust executive management needs to demonstrate a clearer commitment to all midwifery staff and the role of the Professional Midwifery Advocate (PMA). Midwifery may have a smaller number of staff within an NHS Trust, but this does not mean that they should not have a voice on executive management committees, including on issues that affect workplace culture, maintenance of staff numbers (NHS England, 2023b) and provision of high-quality care that is accessible by all.

Reassessment of NIPE practitioners

The *NIPE screening programme handbook* (PHE, 2021a) does discuss updating of staff, which should be an expectation of professional practice. However, in some Trust sites where staff have successfully achieved their NIPE qualification, then are expected to conduct a number of NIPEs still under supervision. This needs to be reviewed, particularly in relation to newly qualified midwives (NQMs) who have trained in the Trust, as there is no valid reason to reassess their competency in this activity when this is not required in terms of their other midwifery activities. If staff have come from another Trust, with a different digital platform, policies and guidelines, then extra support is undoubtedly beneficial. What all NIPE practitioners have stated that they would like is to be supported by a 'buddy system' so that they can gain confidence, information and support when commencing solo practice (Dolby, 2023). The level of support should be related to their background training, if this is a different Trust site or, for example, if they previously worked with different protocols. This type of supportive activity would engender staff well-being instead of making them think that although they have gained a qualification, they are being made to feel incompetent before they have even started independent, autonomous practice.

Although the NIPE programme does not stipulate the number of NIPEs that a practitioner is required to perform each year in order to maintain practical competency, it is prudent to consider the stage of NIPE experience. For example, a practitioner who has just completed the prerequisite training or has had a break in service will require regular participation in the NIPE if they are to embed and hone their skills to a higher level. This only comes with the experience and confidence that develop from regular participation. A practice arena that encourages such development not only helps confidence levels to rise, but also enables those areas of the NIPE, such as the hip examination, that need a high level of competency to be fine-tuned as the practitioner's expertise grows.

The onus is therefore not only on each individual practitioner to recognise their need for consolidation and knowledge, but also for their employers to support staff development and access to areas where skill levels can be further developed to meet and maintain best practice. In relation to NIPE and professional practice, **all** members of the interprofessional team must have the same access to updating and skill development, and respect each other's roles if they are to work together to achieve a high standard of practice, smooth routes of referral, as well as effective parental and professional communication and support.

5 Safeguarding

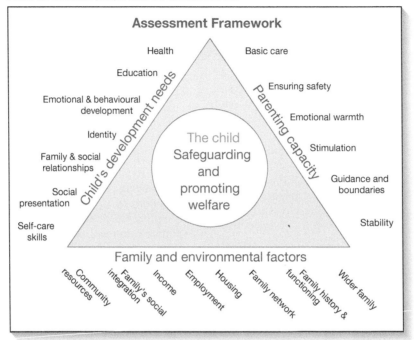

Figure 5.1 Safeguarding assessment framework – the three domains of good assessment.
Source: HM Government (2023)/CROWN COPYRIGHT/CC BY 3.0.

Table 5.1 Safeguarding statistics.

	Referrals	Children in need	Child Protection Plans (CPP)/ Register (CPR)
England	640 430	403 090	50 780 (CPP)
Scotland	11 473	3286	2031 (CPR)
Wales	209 008	46 685	3670 (CPR)
Northern Ireland	35 503	22 875	2171 (CPR)

Source: Department for Education (2023); Scottish Government (2023); Welsh Government (2023); Northern Ireland Department of Health (2023).

Physical Examination of the Newborn at a Glance, Second Edition. Dr Lyn Dolby and Denise (Dee) Campbell.
© 2025 John Wiley & Sons Ltd. Published 2025 by John Wiley & Sons Ltd.

Safeguarding could relate to a vulnerable adult or a child. A pregnant woman may have physical, sensory or mental impairment, or a learning disability increasing their vulnerability. However, when examining the newborn the greater potential for involvement in safeguarding remains with a recognised cause for concern (raised antenatally or in the early post-natal period) and, more particularly, in the preventative health promotion and education shared with the parent during the examination (see Chapters 6 and 7).

Safeguarding is about preventing harm to vulnerable individuals. It is not child protection, which is a response to potential or actual harm. Recent statistics from 2023 identify that 896 414 safeguarding referrals were made to children's social services across the United Kingdom; of those, 475 936 children were identified as 'children in need' and 58 652 required placement on a protection plan (England) or a Child Protection Register (Scotland, Wales and Northern Ireland) (Department for Education, 2023; Scottish Government, 2023; Welsh Government, 2023; Northern Ireland Department of Health, 2023) (Table 5.1).

Safeguarding and promoting the welfare of children (HM Government, 2023, pp. 7–8) is defined as:

- Providing help and support to meet the needs of children as soon as problems emerge.
- Protecting children from maltreatment, whether that is within or outside the home, including online.
- Preventing impairment of children's mental or physical health or development.
- Ensuring that children grow up in circumstances consistent with the provision of safe and effective care.
- Promoting the upbringing of children with their birth parents or family network, through a kinship care arrangement, whenever possible and when this is in the best interest of the children.
- Taking action to enable all children to have the best outcomes as set out in the children's social care national framework (Department for Education, 2024).

Since the Children Act 2004, there has been appreciation of the need for a local duty of responsibility on multi-agency working around safeguarding. The UK Government (HM Government, 2023) provides clarification of the individual legislative requirements as well as understanding of the frameworks for Local Safeguarding Partners (LSPs). LSPs have the role of reviewing safeguarding procedures and the promotion of welfare. They ensure multi-agency and partnership working through a framework involving all three LSPs: the local authority, integrated care boards, and Chief Constable. The guide to multi-agency working should be read in conjunction with any relevant local NHS Trust policies and protocols.

Practitioners performing the physical examination of the newborn have an important role in safeguarding. They offer an early newborn/infant-centred approach in their education of the parent, plus collaboration with numerous partners providing care.

Numerous guidelines exist around factors that may contribute towards the vulnerability of a child. The National Institute for Health and Care Excellence (NICE, 2017a) reminds us to appreciate that circumstances vary and that not all children in vulnerable groups will be affected – neither will every child fit neatly into any one category. The following list pulls together the common issues identified (Birthrights, 2024; ICON, 2023; NICE, 2017a):

- Substance misuse within the family (drug and alcohol).
- Domestic abuse.
- Emotional volatility or anger problems.
- Mental health problems.
- Previous history of personal abuse, child abuse or unexplained child death.
- Non-engagement or non-compliance with health or social services.
- Denial of pregnancy.
- Parent aged under 16 years.
- Age of child.
- Gender – unwanted gender.
- Disability.
- Stressful and overwhelming infant crying.

Protection from maltreatment and the provision of safe care may have required initiation antenatally through the assessment framework (see Figure 5.1). The children's social care (CSC) agencies will accept referrals from the time a fetus reaches 18–20 weeks' gestation, so the decision may already have been taken to place the newborn under local authority care. On every occasion when an examination is carried out, the practitioner must follow local policy and protocols around how to access any database or register associated with social care and check that neither the mother nor the infant has been named there. The plan of care may involve removal of the baby from the parents at birth or prior to leaving the maternity unit, either with parental consent or through a court order. Removal occurs only when evidence of vulnerability is significant enough that there is considered to be an immediate risk:

- Known child protection concerns, possibly linked to a sibling.
- Current criminal status.
- Health or disability concerns preventing parents from providing newborn care even within available support systems.
- Rejection of support systems.

6 Health promotion: information for parents

Physical Examination of the Newborn at a Glance, Second Edition. Dr Lyn Dolby and Denise (Dee) Campbell.
© 2025 John Wiley & Sons Ltd. Published 2025 by John Wiley & Sons Ltd.

Box 6.1 Feeding and elimination.

	Average quantity over 24 h	
Ask parents about the number of wet and dirty nappies over the last 24 hours. The number will depend on the age of the neonate, the method and quantity of feeding and the general condition of the baby.	**1–2 days of age:** wet = 1–2 or more dirty = 1 or more	**5–6 days of age:** wet = 5 or more dirty = 2 or more

Assess colour of urine and stools – see Chapter 32 on Excretion.

Box 6.2 BCG: what you and parents need to know.

- What are the unit protocols in relation to both maternal and neonatal need for BCG vaccination?
- Which babies are at risk and why?
- What actions will you need to take if vaccination is required?
- Have you made an appropriate entry on S4N?

Table 6.1 Safer sleeping/sudden infant death syndrome (SIDS).

Supine position	The baby is placed on their back when asleep. The baby can be placed in the prone position when awake, but when they fall asleep or the parent leaves the room the baby should be placed on their back.
Placement in the cot	Small cribs are not usually an issue, although the cot bedding should still be placed across the baby leaving their arms out. Two layers are normally sufficient and no hat is required. In a larger cot the baby should be moved down to the point where their feet can touch the foot of the cot – this will prevent the baby from wriggling down underneath the bedding and overheating. No cot bumpers or toys should be used.
Breastfeeding	Partial breastfeeding lowers the risk of SIDS, and exclusive breastfeeding is associated with the lowest risk.
Temperature	Room temperature should be approx. 16–20 °C. The baby should be able to maintain a temperature of 36.5–37.5 °C in this room temperature. Most babies are capable of this 6 h after birth and therefore no hat is required indoors. Parents should be shown how to assess temperature in the absence of a digital thermometer.
Smoking	Passive smoking is a factor in SIDS. Parents who smoke should not do so within the rooms where the baby is placed. Ideally, the smoker needs to go outside to smoke, but should be made aware that the chemicals they have inhaled will be exhaled over the next two hours. Removing outer clothing and/or cleaning teeth is not enough to reduce the risk.
Room sharing	Risk of SIDS is reduced when the baby sleeps in their own cot alongside the parental bed for the first 6 months of life. Bed sharing is not advisable, particularly if a parent smokes, has consumed alcohol or 'street drugs' (some are referred to as 'recreational'), is on other medication that affects depth of sleep, is a 'heavy' sleeper or is feeling extremely tired.
ICON	Parents should be made aware of what ICON stands for and that it is OK to walk away from a crying baby (as long as the baby is safe) to breathe, relax and give themselves time to become calm before returning to their baby. Crying babies can be very stressful. See https://iconcope.org for more information.

Source: Adapted from The Lullaby Trust / https://www.lullabytrust.org.uk, last accessed 11 May 2024.

Table 6.2 Signs of neonatal cardiovascular and respiratory dysfunction.

Aspect	Signs
Respiration	Poor (gasping/irregular) or absent
Skin colour and mucous membranes	Pale or dusky (blue/grey) Mucous membranes of the mouth appear blue/very dark red
Tone	Floppy, inactive, poorly flexed
Attentive/responsive	Little recognition of surroundings, even though eyes are open, unresponsive

Part of the newborn examination process is to impart health promotion information to the parents once the findings of the examination have been explained and questions answered. Any interaction between the practitioner and parents during daily care can provide an ideal opportunity to inform parents about their baby's health and development. This includes aspects such as normal neonatal reflexes, hearing and vision. It is also important to visually assess the baby even when not actually performing any form of neonatal examination, for example the darker the neonatal skin colour the more important it becomes to assess for cyanosis and jaundice, and all babies should be assessed for the presence of normal behaviour and movement.

However, the full physical examination of the newborn is a specific opportunity to inform parents about the *key* health and wellbeing aspects that will inform them about their child's initial abilities (including positive parenting – see NHS England, 2021 and UNICEF, 2023) and possible signs of ill health where they may need to seek advice or will need to take immediate action. For some parents, information about access to further support for specific conditions or referral due to issues found during the newborn examination may also be important factors to discuss. Parents need to be given this information at the time of the examination, not later on discharge or via a video clip (the key points may need to be discussed further for clarity). The focus should be on their baby and the information that they need to know in relation to their baby's immediate future.

Key discussion points

Feeding is typically a good place to start, as feeding issues are always a point of discussion. Parents are often tired and sometimes need time to catch up with the fact that the examination itself is over and that they now need to attend to the information they are being given.

A normal output (Box 6.1) will reassure parents that the baby is obtaining adequate supplies of milk, particularly when breastfeeding. Parents need to know that as their baby grows more milk is required and the baby may be unsettled for a period of time. See Chapter 32 to review normal urine excretion, natural stool changes and signs that may be more serious.

Details on **immunisations**, when they commence and where they will be administered needs to be conveyed to parents. They should be informed that information on immunisation is incorporated within the PCHR, as the time for the first vaccination will arrive soon and that they need to know what their decision is. They also need to know if changes have been made since their last child was vaccinated (if this is a second plus child) and if any particular issues are presently arising. For example:

• Parents should be made aware that the incidence of measles is rising (UK Health Security Agency, 2024). Staff need to know the risks of measles in the workplace and about the RCPCH (2023) 'Think Measles' poster, which also gives access to images of the rash on different skin tones by using the QR codes printed on the poster.
• The bacille Calmette–Guérin (BCG) vaccination may be offered at birth if the newborn will travel to (or be visited by relatives from) an area with a high prevalence of tuberculosis. Maternity units will either offer this prior to discharge or refer parents to their GP for the vaccination. See Box 6.2 in relation to what you and parents need to know.

Parents can gain further information from the content included in the PCHR and access the UK Health Security Agency (2023) guide to immunisations, which covers both babies and children.

Car seats and travel systems do not often give enough information about how to use them correctly and why. The car seat should be used for the purpose intended – vehicle travel – as it is purposely restrictive in order to reduce trauma in the event of an accident. Travel systems enabling a car seat to be attached to a pram chassis should be restricted to periods of no longer than two hours of use. Therefore, if a baby is in the seat during a journey and then remains in the seat afterwards, the time for which they are in that one position can be longer than recommended. Due to the restrictive function of the seat, it reduces the movement of the baby, particularly of the hips, and prolonged restriction may affect hip development (see Chapter 49). Removing the baby to a flatbed allows normal leg movement that aids in hip development. Babies who are small or have respiratory issues should not be in a car seat for longer than 30 minutes.

Parents also need to be informed that it is crucial to consider where the seat belts enter the back of the car seat. When the baby is sitting in the seat, the insertion point of the belt in the back of the seat should be clearly visible at the top of the shoulder, but as the baby grows this point of insertion will drop down out of view. This is the moment when the belt needs to be moved to the next higher insertion point, reducing the possibility of trauma caused by poor belt positioning during an accident. Puffy winter coats and blankets should not be used under the seatbelt as they reduce the effectiveness of the belt system.

Safer sleeping can be one of the factors that reduces the risk of sudden infant death syndrome (SIDS). However, the baby's temperature, the risk of passive smoking and how and where the baby is placed to sleep are also factors. Table 6.1 highlights the key points to consider when discussing this subject with parents. Consideration must also be given to providing clear, sensitively portrayed rationales in relation to the information given to parents, as some cultures may practise particular activities that can raise the risk of SIDS. The same sensitivity should be employed for parents who have personal experience of SIDS occurring with one of their children and they will need extra support and information over the coming weeks.

SIDS, 'sudden unexpected death in infancy' (SUDI) and Care of the Next Infant (CONI) will be discussed in Chapter 7. This chapter contains information that professionals need to be conversant with in terms of their own role and actions as well as in relation to the standard of bereavement care that should be provided.

ICON is defined as **I**nfant crying is normal, **C**omforting methods can help, it is **O**K to walk away, **N**ever, ever shake a baby.

ICON aims to help prevent abusive head trauma (AHT) and healthcare staff and parents have access to the website https://icon-cope.org for more information. AHT is a more appropriate term than that often used by the media, 'shaken head syndrome'. There is also growing concern that another form of AHT is starting to occur that is termed 'compressed head syndrome' (Macorano et al., 2023). Future research may be able to highlight the prevalence of this type of abuse.

Discussing **signs of ill health and where to seek advice** provides important pieces information for all parents, whether their baby has been found to have a condition that needs monitoring or treatment, has spent time in a special care baby unit/neonatal intensive care unit or transitional care, or has no apparent issues. The neonatal period is a time for further development of the baby's organs and systems, which can mean that the signs and symptoms of a condition may only become apparent after a period of time. For example, some conditions that cause heart murmurs or jaundice may not be detectable at the time of the newborn examination, but signs will become noticeable later.

Babies can contract harmless infections such as colds and sniffles that provide an important stimulus to their immune system. Parents can discuss these with their midwife, health visitor, GP or practice nurse. However, there are signs of ill health that are more serious and parents should be enabled to recognise these and act appropriately. This is particularly important if these signs relate to poor cardiovascular or respiratory function, as highlighted in Table 6.2. Parents need to know that in this case they should ring for an ambulance, stating how old the baby is and what they are witnessing in their baby.

Parents must be reassured that significant ill health is rare but requires an urgent response. They may be tired and have experienced major changes to their lives, so may not remember every detail you share with them. However, there is growing awareness that when events do occur it is the parents who have been informed about what to watch out for who tend to respond quickest and most appropriately. This in itself is a reason to conduct conversations in relation to health promotion immediately on completion of the newborn examination.

The **next assessment** (infant examination) needs to be highlighted to all parents. As part of the neonatal screening programme, a second physiological assessment (infant examination) is performed at 6 to 8 weeks of age by the GP. This examination aligns with the completed transition from intra- to extrauterine life. Therefore, any congenital condition should have been discovered by this point and the development of the neonate in terms of growth and behaviour should be as expected relevant to post-birth age.

Promoting the health and well-being of the neonate is an important role and should not be underestimated. The information given will increase parental awareness of their child's abilities and future needs and may thus reduce neonatal morbidity and mortality.

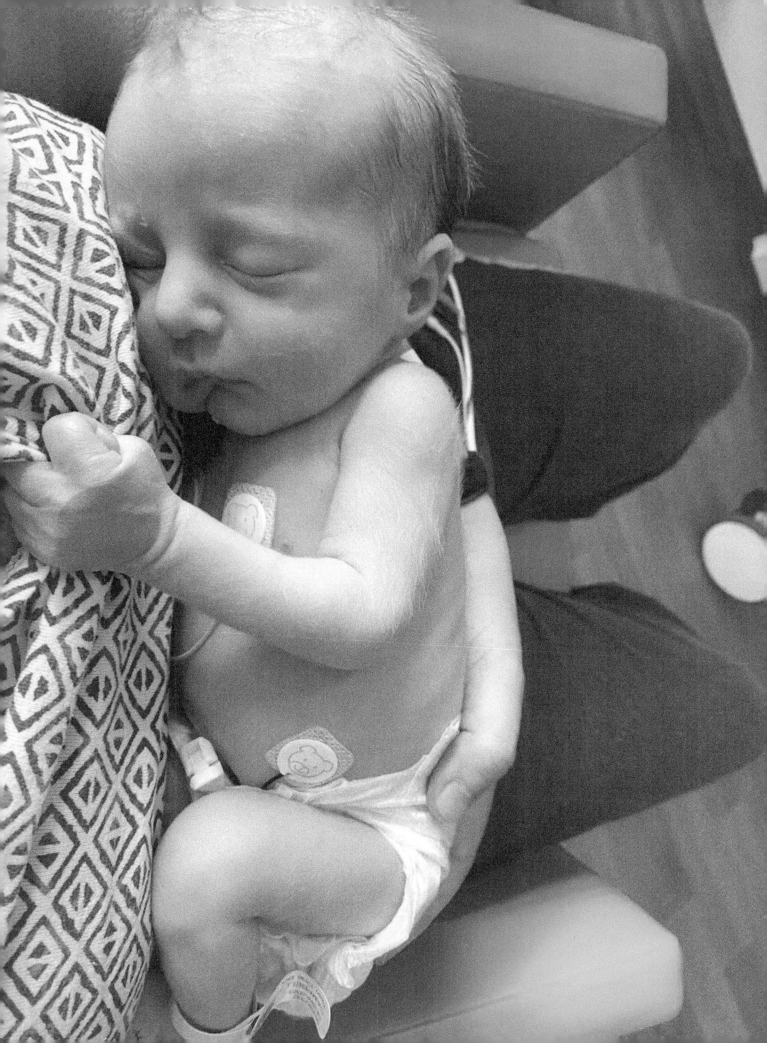

7 Health promotion: additional information for students and practitioners

Box 7.1 National Bereavement Care Pathway definitions.

SUDI	Sudden unexpected death in infancy encompasses all cases in which the death of a baby would not have been reasonably expected in the 24 hours prior to their death and in which no pre-existing medical cause of death is apparent. This is a descriptive term used at the time the baby dies, and will include those deaths for which a cause is ultimately found as well as those that remain unexplained following investigation.
SIDS	Sudden infant death syndrome refers to the sudden and unexpected death of a baby under 12 months of age that remains unexplained after a thorough investigation.

Source: Adapted from RCPCH (2016).

Box 7.2 Office for National Statistics: terms used for census data collection.

Sudden infant death syndrome (SIDS)	Any notification that includes sudden infant death, cot death, SIDS, crib death or other similar term mentioned on the death certificate
Unascertained deaths	Any notification that includes 'other ill-defined and specified causes of mortality', including cases where the only mention on the death certificate is unascertained death
Unexplained infant death	This term includes both SIDS and unascertained death

Figure 7.1 The Lullaby Trust: available information.

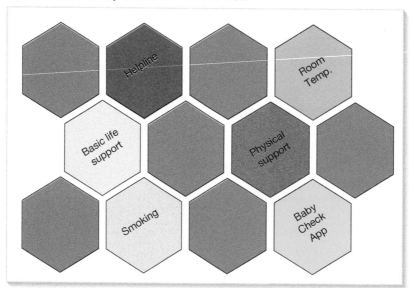

Physical Examination of the Newborn at a Glance, Second Edition. Dr Lyn Dolby and Denise (Dee) Campbell.
© 2025 John Wiley & Sons Ltd. Published 2025 by John Wiley & Sons Ltd.

This chapter highlights particular information that you need to be aware of in relation to SUDI and SIDS.

The National Bereavement Care Pathway (NBCP) developed guidelines for NHS Trusts and staff in relation to improving care for families who experience the loss of a baby (NBCP, 2022). This loss may be due to miscarriage, ectopic or molar pregnancy, termination for fetal anomaly, stillbirth, neonatal death or SUDI up to 12 months. The NBCP developed the guidelines through a multi-agency core group and supported by the Department of Health and Social Care (DHSC) and Teddy's Wish (www.teddyswish.org). NHS England provides learning modules for healthcare staff that are also highlighted within the NBCP guidelines.

The NBCP (2022) uses the definitions as highlighted within the Kennedy Guidelines (RCPCH, 2016; see Box 7.1). However, both students and practitioners need to take care when reading the available literature or a parent's prior notes, so that they are clear on their understanding of the terms used (Pease et al., 2023). For example, statistics within the census publications issued by the Office of National Statistics that relate to unexplained death in infancy also use particular terms when data gathering from death certificates for their current census round (see Box 7.2).

Unexplained infant mortality

A total of 166 unexplained infant deaths (aged birth to one year) occurred in England and Wales in 2021. These account for 7.1% of all infant deaths and continue to be more likely in males before the age of four months and in low-birthweight babies. This rate is lower than the figures for 2011 (244 unexplained infant deaths), but according to the Office for National Statistics (ONS, 2023) the rate remains steady with slight rises and falls. However, it is important to note that the statistics only include those notified in the year of data release. Therefore, due to the delays during the Coronavirus pandemic the exact data will not become clear until the next census is released, when late notifications will be available and will be used to update the current figures. Another source of information that practitioners can access in relation to newborn health and child mortality is Odd et al. (2023).

Unexplained mortality is still in general related to infants born to mothers under 20 years of age (0.95 deaths per 1000 live births) and is lowest in mothers aged 35–39 years of age (0.14 deaths per 1000 live births). However, healthcare professionals should read the current census to appreciate which groups of the population may be at higher risk so that they are better informed as to how to support families where infants may be perceived at higher risk (Pease et al., 2023). It should be noted that such mortality may occur unconnected with any risk factor.

It is generally perceived that accessible information and professional explanation regarding safer sleeping practices, plus the decrease in maternal smoking (NHS, 2022), have aided in the decline in the death rate since 2014. This may further signify the need for health professionals to provide parents with clear information at the time of the NIPE, when parents are often responsive to listening and asking questions about their baby.

Care of the next baby

An understanding of the NBCP (NBCP, 2022) and the investigatory procedures that occur after a sudden infant death can enable staff to have a better understanding of the experiences of parents. Likewise, an understanding of how to support parents with their next infant can greatly help them during a time when they may be worried about the next infant's survival. Guilt may be experienced due to the death of their last infant and they may be concerned about how they will be perceived as parents. Practitioners need to discuss with parents the support available. They also need to be particularly mindful that post-traumatic stress can also be a prevalent feature (NHS England, 2019).

Some NHS Trusts have adopted the Care of the Next Infant programme (CONI), which can help families during the pregnancy and birth and after birth by providing positive support. The Lullaby Trust (2020) provides a booklet for parents and other sources of information that identify what may be available in terms of assistance, equipment and actions they can undertake (see Figure 7.1). The Lullaby Trust has alluded to the need for parents to be aware that not all actions or available equipment are suitable for all families, which enables parents to develop a realistic understanding that may better inform their decision making throughout the journey of bringing a new infant into their lives.

8 Communication during the examination

Figure 8.1 Communication during the examination.

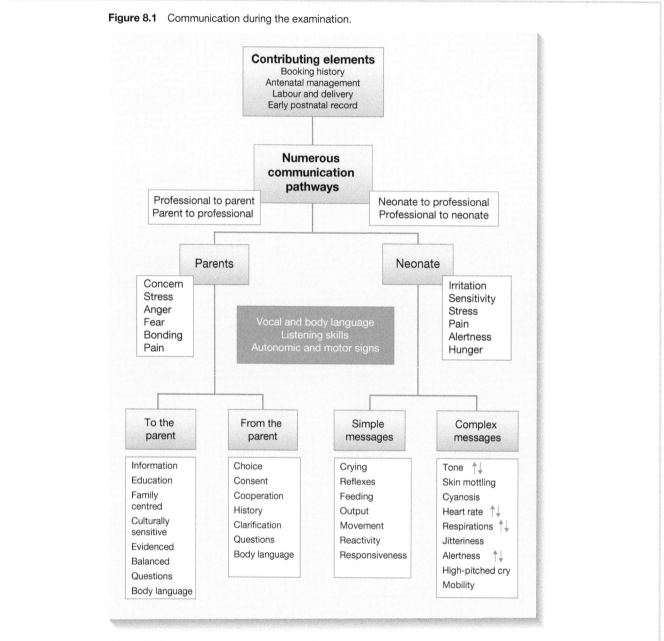

Physical Examination of the Newborn at a Glance, Second Edition. Dr Lyn Dolby and Denise (Dee) Campbell.
© 2025 John Wiley & Sons Ltd. Published 2025 by John Wiley & Sons Ltd.

The numerous communication pathways that need to be considered during the NIPE are expanded on in this chapter. An introductory overview can be seen in Figure 8.1. Analysis of the full history and management to date will inform the examination. Be aware that not all mothers can offer the family history of the male genetics (e.g. rape victims, some assisted pregnancies, women with multiple partners) and this should be treated sensitively in any discussion.

Communicating with the neonate

Communication with the neonate may seem an unusual aspect to encourage. Here the practitioner is not seeking consent nor attempting a verbal conversation. This is about 'hearing' the messages expressed through the body language, movements and noises made by the neonate. These may relate to a psychological state or a physical condition through alertness, irritability, sensitivity, comfort, stress and even pain.

Every neonate is individual and will demonstrate varying amounts of irritation, sensitivity and stress during the examination. Often there will be obvious predisposing factors linked to the behaviour, such as a hungry baby who is difficult to console. The practitioner should always be alert to those forms of communication that are less readily explained and indicate a need for further screening or diagnostic consideration. This may be a sound such as a hoarse, weak or high-pitched cry. It may be a physical sign of distress, linked to a particular movement or aspect of the examination.

Irritation, sensitivity, stress and pain may be displayed through single aspects such as crying or a more complex system of autonomic and motor signs that may include skin mottling or reddening; increased respiration; jerky movements; arching or unusual stretching of limbs; high-pitched cries; jitteriness, startles or tremors. Similarly, immobility, flaccidity, uneven body tone and a lack of response to stimuli are also worrying 'messages' indicating a decreased level of alertness and responsiveness.

It is important that the practitioner understands the messages from the neonate and alters their management of the examination accordingly. In most cases this will not be an unhealthy baby and it will be the examination itself that is causing irritation, overstimulation or stress. Early awareness of the signs and a change in approach are both for the neonate's comfort and so that the examination can be completed.

Simple things like moving the neonate from under a direct light source; placing a warm hand gently on their head; covering the abdomen with clothing; applying or removing eye contact; gentle rocking or allowing a rest period; and talking gently or keeping quiet can all be considered. Sometimes it may be necessary to postpone the examination until after the more immediate needs (such as feeding) have been satisfied. This is also an opportunity to share information with the parents – to help them understand their baby's communications through observation of the individual behaviours.

Communicating with the parents

Information gleaned from the obstetric, paediatric and midwifery records informs the physical examination but requires confirmation, clarification and enlarging on. Family-centred communications involve full awareness of body language, good listening skills and the ability to explain, detail and balance the information shared. These general principles must also include ensuring that the mother is comfortable and feels able to give her concentration to the conversation. Some individuals may require additional support arranged, such as those with sensory impairment, learning disability, specific language needs or mental health issues.

Person-centred care will demonstrate sensitivity, respect and the necessary adjustments to support cultural differences. Culturally appropriate care must demonstrate skills and knowledge that value ethnicity, nationality, religion, sexuality, gender and diversity (including physical and mental health). This can be enhanced through a willingness to listen, managing personal reactions, non-judgmental attitudes, diplomacy and a genuine desire to achieve mutual trust (Care Quality Commission, 2024).

Personal informed choice and consent

The examination cannot be started or continued without the personal informed choice of the parent and their cooperation throughout (UK National Screening Committee, 2023). This begins with introductions and an explanation of the necessary qualifications. Opportunities must be given for the parents to raise concerns, ask questions and share further details. A balanced approach will share evidence about the benefits and risks and should include details on the following:

- **Process** – head to toe; opportunistic; health promotion.
- **Timing** – before 72 hours/6–8 weeks; between feeds; time taken.
- **Components** – where; what is examined; use of equipment.
- **Limitations** – false positives/negatives; aspects not included; ongoing neonatal development limiting results.
- **Risks** – possible stress; positive result; emergency management.
- **Outcomes** – apparently healthy; referral; further screening or diagnostic review; management of any identified condition.
- Further sources of information available.

If a parent declines part, or all, of the newborn element of the NIPE, this is documented on the NIPE national IT system, neonatal notes and PCHR. The GP and health visitor should be informed. If the later infant element of the NIPE is also declined this is additionally recorded in the GP IT system.

Clarification and ongoing communications

A full review of the notes should have taken place. This is an opportunity to check the accuracy of understanding; to ensure nothing is missing or has changed; and to facilitate the parents sharing any concerns. The practitioner should use their communication skills to ask appropriately detailed questions and identify any evasive body language where supportive prompting may help. Specific questions should be asked to ascertain if any known first-degree relative or sibling has a history of any congenital abnormalities, including heart or renal defects, developmental dysplasia of the hips or visual problems. Be aware of the sensitivity of any information shared.

Throughout the examination the communication should be two way. While it is important to take opportunities as they arise to share information on health promotion and parenting skills, it should not become a 'lecture' from the practitioner (no matter how well intentioned). Individualise questions and information sharing and allow time for any replies – take time to listen to what is said as well as observing body language cues.

It is important to appreciate that the parents are also listening intently to all they hear and watching body language too. Beware of using unfamiliar words without explaining their meaning. Ensure that parents are not given cause for alarm where none exists – for example, explain about listening to the baby's heart in various places and for up to a minute. At the end of the examination explain all results sensitively, including any further care required.

9 Communicating concerns to parents

Figure 9.1 Communicating concerns to parents.

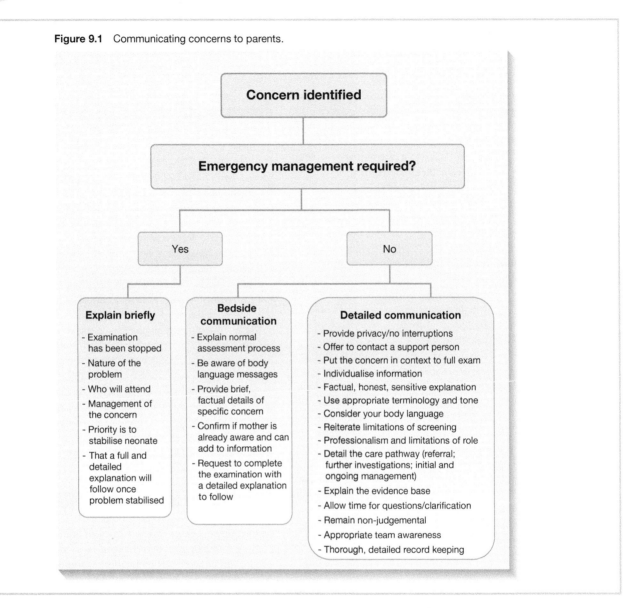

Physical Examination of the Newborn at a Glance, Second Edition. Dr Lyn Dolby and Denise (Dee) Campbell.
© 2025 John Wiley & Sons Ltd. Published 2025 by John Wiley & Sons Ltd.

Inevitably there will be occasions when the examination identifies either a potential, or actual, physical abnormality or concern. If this is an emergency situation, then the examination is stopped and immediate management of the concern is required. However, in most situations the examination can continue to allow all further information to be gleaned and included in the full analysis of the neonate's condition (Figure 9.1).

Be aware that even the most skilful practitioner will often give away clues to a problem through their body language, even when the smallest of concerns is identified. While some information may need to be shared immediately, it is essential to explain that a fully completed examination is required to determine the true extent of any problem and to ensure there are no further problems identified. The parents will not appreciate a 'changing story' in which the problem described initially is found later to be less of an issue. Neither will they maintain their confidence in a practitioner when the picture described is continually changing, or worsening as the examination progresses.

There must be full appreciation of the need for delicacy around information sharing. This includes the terminology and intonation used, as well as the involvement of supportive body language. Time must be allowed for understanding. This balance of communications will ensure that it is not just 'what is said' but also 'how it is said' that will support the parents.

Be prepared for questions and some anxiety from the parents. Answer the questions factually and with honesty, but taking care to avoid assumptions and generalisations. In most cases it is advisable to reiterate the benefits of finishing the examination before all questions can be answered, so that all the relevant factors can be screened for and a full understanding of the concern be known. This prevents the sharing of misleading information; reduces the risk of causing undue worry; and gives the mother some time to digest that there is a problem. Plus it allows an opportunity to move to a more private area for the discussion where the likelihood of disturbance is minimised.

Appreciate personal limitations and do not cross professional boundaries. Be honest about the limits of your expertise and share with the parents any involvement to be expected from more senior or specialist practitioners. This may even include a personal lack of experience in breaking bad news – in which case arranging for a more experienced colleague to join the information sharing may benefit the parents too. It may be appropriate to reiterate information around false-positive results specific to the current concern and to detail the care pathway that will now be followed. This should include specific information around any referral to be made (to whom, when and how), as well as any further screening or diagnostic investigations to be requested (by whom, when and what this will entail). Consider if any senior paediatric referral should be expedited to reduce stress for parents around waiting times. This is often more feasible for the first examination when the mother and baby are still within inpatient care.

The practitioner should be aware of the possible impact of any bad news and of approaches that can be used to reasonably limit distress. Time should be taken to seek assurances that the mother understands the degree of the problem, but this must be with awareness that every parent will react differently. While the examination may only have revealed a medically insignificant problem, each parent brings to the discussion various factors that will influence their degree of reaction and this can be both positive and negative. For example, if antenatal screening has introduced the possibility of a severe abnormality being present, then news of a more minor one will be received positively. However, identifying the same minor concern where there was no prior awareness can be devastating for new parents. Additionally, the mother may have any number of aspects affecting both her ability to disseminate the information shared and how she responds. New parenthood is not always a time of joy: emotions can be affected by being post-operative, sleep deprived or in pain, let alone being negatively affected by transitional hormones or having socio-economic worries. Cultural, ethnic and social issues may also affect the initial responses and outward display of emotion. It is important that your communication remains non-judgemental of any reaction received.

If there is any interim management or aspects of ongoing care that the neonate will benefit from, the parents need to be made aware of these and supported to be involved in providing this care. This may involve monitoring feeding (e.g. during periods of jaundice) or changes to nappy care routines (e.g. when developmental dysplasia of the hip is suspected).

It may be appropriate to offer to contact the husband/partner or an alternative family member/friend if they are not with the mother at the time of the examination. The practitioner should then return when they have arrived to explain the findings of the examination and answer any further questions. Even when both parents were present initially, it is likely that they will have further questions and aspects to discuss after the initial information has been absorbed.

Coping with anger or aggression

In some rare cases the reaction of one or more of the parents will involve anger or aggression. Dealing with bad news can be influenced by the physiological response of the body to the fears brought on by the bad news – a 'fight or flight' reaction. This may also be about the individuals' educational level, prior social learning and a lack of alternative coping strategies. Additionally, attempts to cope may lead to self-preservation actions and wanting to apportion blame. There may also be contributing factors that make this particularly likely, for instance if there have already been concerns expressed around antenatal or labour management or a delayed/difficult delivery, which the parents may now feel is to blame.

In the majority of cases the aggression will be minor, non-physical and will diffuse just as quickly as it occurred. When this is not the case, the practitioner should employ approaches to both guarantee their own safety and help to diffuse the situation. Initially there may be a benefit in allowing the parents an opportunity to express their views and opinions. This may allow a better understanding of their exact concerns and perhaps inform the practitioner how to help. When responding, maintain a calm voice, speak quietly and adopt a non-threatening body posture with relaxed arms and lowered eyes (directed at chin height). If there is any risk of physical aggression, withdraw from the situation and employ team support. In extreme cases it may also be necessary to consider the safety of other adults in proximity as well as the neonate. The practitioner should apply Trust policies for dealing with aggression towards themselves or others.

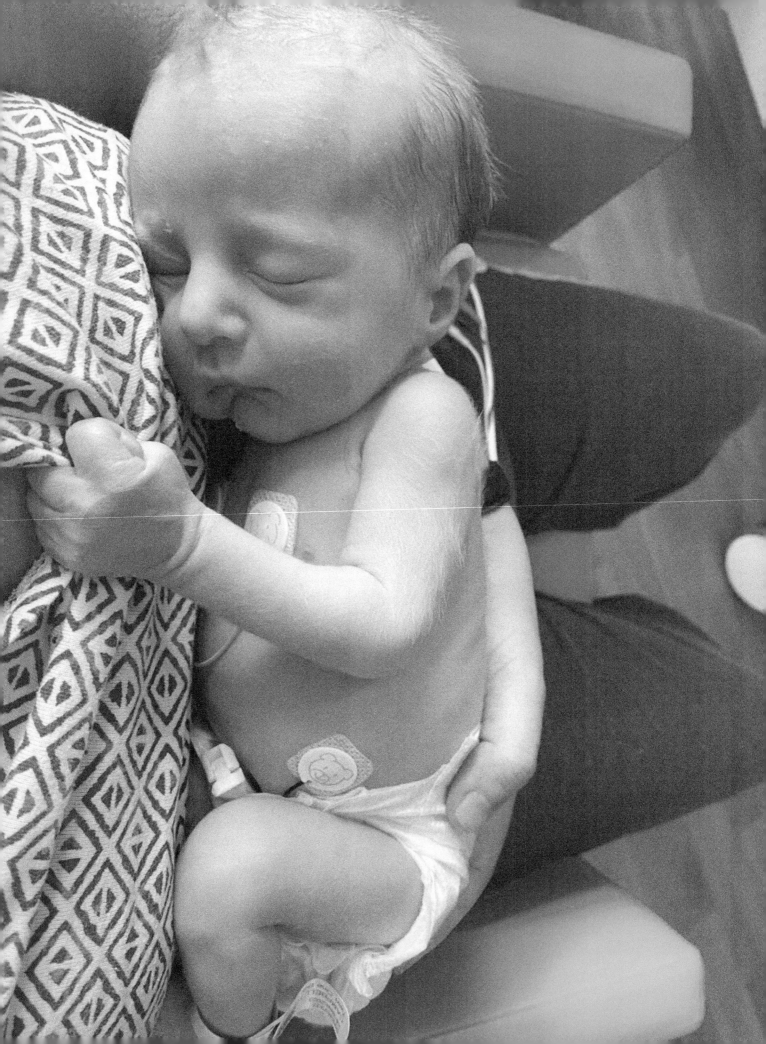

Neonatal physiology and pathophysiology

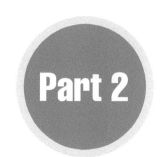

Part 2

Chapters

10 Adaptation to neonatal life: in utero

Figure 10.1   The normal fetal and newborn heart.

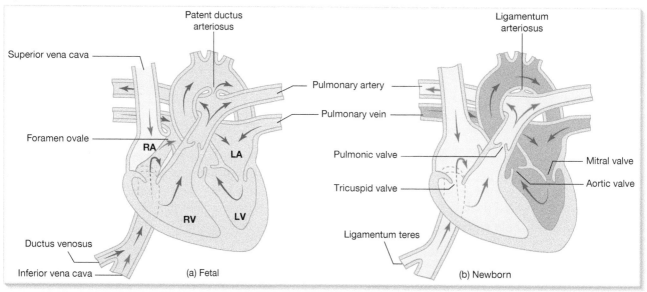

Table 10.1   The three key structures involved in fetal to neonatal adaptation.

Structure	Role
Ductus venosus	'Venosus' – a shunt connecting vein to vein Carries blood with a high oxygen content (80% O_2) from the placenta through the fetal abdominal wall Shunts blood directly to the inferior vena cava Regulates blood flow via a sphincter that closes when blood flow in the umbilical vein reduces and stops When no longer in use, deposition of connective tissue within the duct lumen causes its closure, forming the ligamentum venosum
Foramen ovale	A flap (opening left to right) in the septum between the right and left atria Shunts high O_2 concentration blood from areas of high pressure to low pressure Closes when pulmonary resistance decreases as blood is sent to the lungs; decreased pressure on the right side of heart with a corresponding increased pressure on the left side of the heart Initial closure is caused by the pressure changes keeping the flap functionally closed until deposition of fibrous tissue creates a permanent closure, the fossa ovalis
Ductus arteriosus	Shunts blood from pulmonary artery to aorta Protective function: damage to fetal lungs could occur in the event of circulatory overload Enables strengthening of the right ventricle Carries medium O_2 saturated blood Development is influenced by maternal prostaglandin levels and resistance created by non-functioning lungs Closes when prostaglandin levels start to diminish, lungs expand and resistance is reduced; O_2 levels become elevated Bradykinin also assists in duct closure in the presence of high O_2 levels. It is released by lungs on inflation and acts to contract the smooth muscle of the duct Constricts from birth, usually closes fully within the first 24–48 h of life – results in ligamentum arteriosus

Table 10.2   Changes from fetal to adult structures.

Fetal structure	Adult structure
Ductus venosus	Ligamentum venosum
Foramen ovale	Fossa ovalis
Ductus arteriosus	Ligamentum arteriosus
Umbilical vein	Ligamentum teres
Umbilical arteries and abdominal ligaments	Medial umbilical ligaments Superior vesicular artery (supplies the bladder)

Physical Examination of the Newborn at a Glance, Second Edition. Dr Lyn Dolby and Denise (Dee) Campbell.
© 2025 John Wiley & Sons Ltd. Published 2025 by John Wiley & Sons Ltd.

A complex chain of physiological events commences that enables the fetus to make the transition from intrauterine to extrauterine life. Most fetuses will make the journey into the outside world with little effect from the episodes of mild hypoxaemia that they may experience during labour. However, in the event of cardiorespiratory depression at birth, prompt recognition and effective resuscitation are paramount (see Chapter 13). Figure 10.1 gives a diagrammatic representation of blood flow within the fetal and newborn heart structure.

Fetal respiratory and cardiovascular development

Preparation for active use of the lungs occurs in the fetus from 10 weeks' gestation, when breathing movements start to occur even though the lung tissue has minimal blood flow and the lungs are in a state of collapse. At approximately 24 weeks' gestation, the secretion of surfactant (a surface-active lipoprotein) commences and begins to coat the internal lining, reducing surface tension. The presence of surfactant enables easier initial lung expansion at birth and aids effective lung function post birth. Also, while in utero the lungs contain roughly 50 mL of fluid, by birth this volume has already started to decrease and approximately 25% of this fluid volume will be expelled via the trachea during birth. By 3 weeks' gestation, the fetal cardiovascular system has started to develop and in the absence of any factors that may interfere with physiological progression (see Chapter 44), normal fetal respiratory and cardiovascular development will continue throughout pregnancy.

In the fetus the source of oxygen is the placenta, which enables the blood arriving via the two umbilical arteries to become oxygenated. This oxygenated blood is then carried to the fetal heart by the umbilical vein, where it is pumped round the fetus and eventually back to the heart to be returned once more to the placenta for oxygenation. The ductus arteriosus, foramen ovale and ductus venosus act to reduce blood flow to the lungs while enabling the majority of oxygenated blood to pass to the major organs (Table 10.1). Only a small amount of oxygenated blood is required by the lungs to allow growth and development in readiness for extrauterine life.

Fetal to neonatal adaptation

Preparation for effective lung expansion is encouraged by the creation of a negative intrathoracic pressure and an increased external atmospheric pressure alongside an accelerated production of surfactant in order to inhibit atelectasis. At birth, two-thirds of the lung liquid has already been expelled or is absorbed into the neonatal bloodstream or lymphatics within a few minutes of birth. The change in temperature (from warm uterine environment to the cooler outside air) and the physical stimulus of light, touch and sound cause the central nervous system to react. Chemical stimulus in the form of dramatic increases in the levels of serum cortisol, anti-diuretic hormone (ADH), thyroid-stimulating hormone (TSH) and catecholamines (neurotransmitters) serve to initiate breathing. Anthony and McKinlay (2022) give a good overview of the physiology of fetal adaptation to extrauterine life.

Occlusion of the umbilical cord effectively closes down the low pressure exerted by the placenta. With the first gasp the lungs expand and pulmonary vascular resistance is further reduced as the pulmonary vessels dilate, increasing arterial oxygen tension. As a result, systemic vascular resistance increases and reducing blood flow to the ductus venosus causes it to constrict within minutes of birth. Deposition of connective tissue within the entire ductus lumen starts within days after birth, with permanent structural closure usually being completed by 1–3 months of age.

The increased pulmonary circulation raises the pressure in the left atrium, forcing the septum primum against the septum secundum, thus causing the gradual closure of the foramen ovale. However, functional closure brought about by proliferation of fibrous tissue will not occur for some days, allowing some mixing of oxygenated and deoxygenated blood to occur. If the condition of coarctation of the aorta occurs, steroidal therapy should be used to prevent functional closure of the foramen ovale and enable continuation of the mixing of oxygenated and deoxygenated blood. Fetal respiratory and cardiovascular development can buy some time for the neonate until surgical treatment can be performed.

The ductus arteriosus acts as a shunt from the descending aorta to the left pulmonary artery near the bifurcation of the pulmonary trunk. During fetal life, the low PaO_2 and the vasodilatory effect of circulating prostaglandins (PGE2) maintain the patency of the duct. However, after birth, when pulmonary oxygen saturation increases and circulatory PGE2 reduces, this shunt closes. In the term neonate this closure usually occurs within the first 24–48 hours of life. Permanent closure occurs due to fibrosis of the shunt, which takes 4–6 weeks to complete, and this remnant of fetal life is then referred to as the ligamentum arteriosum. See Table 10.2 for a precis regarding the outcome for fetal structures no longer required post birth.

11 Adaptation to neonatal life at birth: further insight

Table 11.1 Impact of delayed cord clamping on adaptation.

Delayed cord clamping (≥30–60 secs)	
Late pre-term (>32 weeks' gestation) and term neonates	Extra blood transfer increases haemoglobin level, which may reduce the risk of iron deficiency occurring by 3–6 months post birth Higher levels of brain myelin (associated with visual, sensory and motor ability)
Very pre-term neonates (≤32 weeks' gestation)	Can reduce the risk of hypotension, use of inotropes and red cell transfusion, which in turn may enhance survival

Note: In very pre-term neonates (<28 weeks' gestation) intact cord milking is not recommended due to the increased risk of intraventricular haemorrhage.

Table 11.2 Persistent pulmonary hypertension of the newborn (PPHN).

PPHN is also defined as persistent fetal circulation
Relatively rare but needs to be recognised and managed in a timely manner as it is potentially life-threatening
Caused by either a right-to-left ductal or atrial shunt persisting post birth or   when both occur in the presence of elevated right ventricular pressure
Can be idiopathic but predisposing conditions include intrauterine hypoxia and ischaemia, respiratory distress syndrome, meconium aspiration syndrome, overwhelming sepsis and/or neonatal hypoxia and ischaemia
Can result in severe hypoxaemia, which may lead to increased levels of morbidity and mortality

Reduction in incidence and impact has been due to:
  better understanding and earlier recognition of the condition
  improvements within antenatal and neonatal care
  stringent monitoring of oxygen levels and blood pressure
  prudent use of surfactant therapy

Table 11.3 Activities that support neonatal adaptation post birth.

Event	Result	Action
Over-stimulus	Raised stress levels, increased need for oxygen and glucose, fall in temperature	Dimly lit, warm, quiet birthing room where the baby remains with the parents Immediate skin to skin if parents agree
Inadequate drying of baby at birth	A wet baby soon becomes cold Cold babies increase their use of oxygen and glucose and non-shivering thermogenesis in a bid to maintain body temperature level	Adequately dry baby, put on a hat Skin to skin allows for transference of parental heat to baby Feeding produces heat due to the action of feeding, supplies nutrition to aid glucose levels etc.
Need for mild resuscitation?	Can raise stress levels for both mother and baby, which leads to a greater need for oxygen and glucose Separation of baby from mother may occur	Mild resuscitation can occur while the cord remains unclamped, which is beneficial for the baby Warmth and the inherent stabilisation of cardiac and respiratory ability are enhanced when the baby is directly next to the mother

Note: Pre-term or small for gestational age babies may not have enough brown fat or glucose reserves to instigate or continue to employ physiological measures to maintain cardiac and respiratory function. Hypothermia will only exacerbate the issue.

Neonatal adaptation: supportive activities

It is always worth reviewing how delayed cord clamping can assist in adaptation to extra-uterine life (Rabe et al., 2019). Table 11.1 gives a few key reasons for delaying cord clamping (Anthony and McKinlay, 2022), although it should be borne in mind that the condition of the baby at birth may predispose to cord clamping much earlier. The Resuscitation Council UK (2021a) also advocates a delay in cord clamping (a least 60 seconds) when immediate higher-level resuscitation or stabilisation is not required, such as in some congenital heart conditions, sepsis or persistent pulmonary hypertension of the newborn (PPHN; see the overview of PPHN in Table 11.2).

Physiological management in relation to the delivery of the placenta needs to be a subject of discussion with the parents prior to the commencement of the labour process, once labour is established and prior to delivery. Parents need to be aware that this management of placental delivery automatically requires no cord clamping and if labour and delivery have occurred 'physiologically', then the third stage of labour can follow the same process. However, this should be reconsidered if circumstances and risk factors for physiological placental delivery, such as maternal anaemia, prolonged labour, augmentation or induction of labour arise, as a uterus unable to commence the process of involution postpartum or low clotting ability in the mother could result in postpartum haemorrhage. Parents should also be informed that a 'physiological' management of the third stage does not usually take any longer than in 'active' management. It is the responsibility of the healthcare professionals to give correct information to the parents so that they can make an informed decision.

It should also be noted that delayed cord clamping in relation to the optimum time period for the delay has been investigated since Rabe et al. (2019) and remains ongoing. Likewise, there is still an ongoing debate in relation to whether the neonate requires vitamin K if the maternal and neonatal clotting and fibrinolytic systems are activated during the process of labour. Therefore, it will be interesting to see the outcome of well-conducted research in the future. However, in the latter case it should be noted that the administration of vitamin K varies across the United Kingdom and that in some Trust sites there is more than one choice available. Therefore parents need to have sufficient information well before administration may occur in order to make an informed decision.

Birthing room activities

Neonatal physiological adaptation can be supported by the activities of those within the birthing environment. Simple measures that reduce stress on both parent and baby can aid the continuation of the transition to extrauterine life so that the baby's physiological functions can stabilise and therefore energy usage is productive and sustaining. Table 11.3 gives a summary of some of the activities that can support a neonate by reducing stress, overstimulus and heat loss.

The neonatal temperature is not stable at birth as the baby has to metabolise glucose stores (non-shivering thermogenesis) in order to create heat (Anthony and McKinlay, 2022). Therefore, if the baby cools, has reduced glucose stores or an infection, it can be difficult for the baby to maintain effective metabolic and oxygen levels, which may compromise well-being. The baby can generate heat through non-shivering thermogenesis, but this also requires increased consumption of glucose and oxygen. If the baby continues to become chilled, their oxygen usage may exceed that of the levels available in air. As a result, metabolic acidosis can occur and the baby may show signs of cyanosis and tachypnoea. If the baby continues to be compromised and becomes hypoglycaemic, constriction of the pulmonary vessels and reduced surfactant levels can lead to respiratory distress. Neonatal physiology may try to address this situation by re-opening the foramen ovale, re-creating the right-to-left shunt and ensuing PPHN.

Continuous assessment of fetal to neonatal adaptation is important to enable the early recognition of conditions or circumstances that may interfere with this process, such as a neonate smaller than expected for the gestational age, infection, antenatal risk factors and other anomalies that may compromise neonatal health.

Over-stimulus is reduced within dimly lit, warm, quiet rooms where the baby remains with the parent and (if they agree) immediate skin-to-skin contact can be instigated. This enables the baby to stabilise temperature, respiratory and cardiac function more quickly. Inability to stabilise these vital functions can result in higher oxygen and glucose needs, which could lead to hypoxia, hypothermia and hypoglycaemia as the baby's organs are immature and will not be able to accommodate adequately. Adequate drying of the baby, use of a hat and being placed skin to skin, plus access to maternal colostrum, will also assist in reducing loss of heat and stabilisation of the baby's core temperature.

12 Thermoregulation, cold stress and hypothermia

Figure 12.1 A simplified representation of the energy triangle.

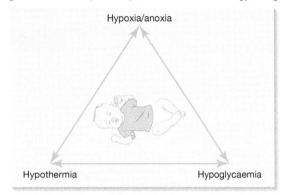

Hypoxia/anoxia

Hypothermia   Hypoglycaemia

Table 12.2 Assessing neonatal temperature with a digital thermometer.

Action	Rationale
Armpit should be dry	Allows good apposition of skin to thermometer tip as dampness can affect the reading
Place the tip of the thermometer under the arm with the thermometer parallel to the body	Good positioning ensures that the tip is not 'poking' into the baby's armpit but enabling good contact with the skin layers
Baby's arm should be brought into contact with the body	Enables effective skin contact by ensuring the probe tip is well covered and prevents surrounding air from affecting the temperature reading

Table 12.1 Environmental heat loss.

Routes	How heat is lost from the body	Prevention
Evaporation	Liquid on the skin of a wet baby and through respiration evaporates into the air	Adequate drying of the skin due to large body surface area Dress in warm clothes and hat
Conduction	Warmth from the baby is transferred to a cooler surface due to poor insulation provided by insufficient layer of neonatal subcutaneous fat	Warm surfaces and clothing, skin to skin with parents
Convection	Air currents take heat away from the skin surface	Turn off fans, close windows and doors to prevent draughts, adequate clothing/hat
Radiation	Heat moves away from the body	Maintain room temperature at 16–20 °C Adequate clothing/bedding/hat

Table 12.3 Neonatal response to cold stress.

Event	Neonatal activity
Peripheral vasoconstriction	Reduces heat lost via the extremities by decreasing the amount of blood within the circulatory system passing through the extremities
Increased heat production	Increases metabolic rate *but* this also necessitates a rise in oxygen consumption and if the fetus developed hypoxia in utero this may reduce the efficiency of this action
Increased voluntary and involuntary muscular activity 'shivering'	Shivering in pre-term infants is non-existent and in term infants the ability to shiver is extremely limited Hypoxia and resultant acidosis in utero will have an impact on this ability particularly when glucose levels may not be in plentiful supply, because of the natural initial reduction in levels soon after birth or due to an inborn error of metabolism, leading to further adverse impact
Non-shivering thermogenesis	During the last trimester of pregnancy, brown adipose tissue (BAT) is deposited primarily around the neck, axilla, scapulae, sternum, adrenals and the kidneys of the fetus. BAT is a highly specialised type of adipose tissue that is well vascularised and the cells are densely packed with mitochondria, which are the power houses behind cellular activity and the provision of energy

Physical Examination of the Newborn at a Glance, Second Edition. Dr Lyn Dolby and Denise (Dee) Campbell.
© 2025 John Wiley & Sons Ltd. Published 2025 by John Wiley & Sons Ltd.

Normal core body temperature is usually classified as 36.5–37.4 °C, whereas a temperature of 34–36.4 °C is viewed as mild hypothermia and 32–35.9 °C as severe hypothermia. Due to the negative impact of cold stress on a newborn infant, it is important to protect the baby from heat loss (Table 12.1). A healthy term baby should be able to regulate their temperature within 6 hours after birth, which is why a hat is often removed near to this time. However, a baby who is pre-term, underweight or otherwise compromised will soon be affected by cold stress if temperature management is inadequate. Neonatal hypothermia is preventable in the newborn and it is not a complication of prematurity or compromise; rather, it is the result of inadequate attention to thermal management (Kyokan et al., 2023). Neonatal temperature assessment can be managed through simple measures (Table 12.1) at the time of birth and the use of appropriate equipment, such as a digital thermometer, that is applied correctly (see Table 12.2). However, research is at present reviewing the effectiveness of infrared thermography (IRT), which enables temperature to be measured from a distance without being invasive and perhaps provides a better understanding of the mechanisms involved in brown adipose tissue (BAT) in neonates (González-García et al., 2022).

Heat management in utero

In utero the fetus has no need for thermoregulation within the warm confines of the uterus (usually a constant 0–5 °C above maternal temperature). However, at birth the immaturity of the thermoregulatory system does not allow for adult reactions to cold such as shivering. Therefore, when birth is imminent, quick assessment of the birthing room environment and the necessary preparation for the baby's arrival (warm towels and clothing etc.) should take place. The activities highlighted in Table 12.1 should aim to reduce the neonatal need to waste valuable oxygen and glucose in the effort to maintain core body temperature.

Neonatal heat management in response to temperature loss

When a neonate is externally protected from temperature loss, oxygen and glucose consumption for thermoregulation remains minimal. However, when heat is lost in the unprotected neonate, they must respond to the cold stress (Table 12.3) and protect themselves in order to survive. Unfortunately, a neonate has immature bodily systems and is unable to gain food or warmth for themselves, and when the usual metabolic defence mechanisms that use oxygen and glucose are exhausted the result is hypothermia (neonatal cold injury).

Hypothermia (neonatal cold injury)

Hypothermia is one of the three major considerations within the 'energy triangle' (Figure 12.1). The close relationship between hypothermia, hypoglycaemia and hypoxia/anoxia must never be under-estimated and understanding the interactions between these three factors and the impact on the newborn baby is paramount. The midwife needs to recognise when intrapartum compromise has occurred and be vigilant in assessing and facilitating the baby's adaptation to extrauterine life and thermal regulation. Aylott (2006) still supplies one of the better explanations as to the importance of understanding how impact on the energy triangle can seriously detract from neonatal health.

Both oxygen consumption and utilisation of glucose will be increased in the event of prolonged exposure to cold and this leads to increasing levels of hypoxia and hypoglycaemia. Peripheral cyanosis will occur in an attempt to maintain core body temperature. Initially the neonate may have been vocally signalling their discomfort, but as the baby becomes colder, lethargy and an unwillingness to feed will soon become evident. If the condition continues unrecognised, the neonate may develop apnoeic spells, which further reduce oxygen levels and exacerbate respiratory distress syndrome. On re-warming the baby's physiological response to the improvement in blood pressure and perfusion is to wash out the products of anaerobic metabolism into the circulation, thereby causing metabolic acidosis. Hypoglycaemia occurs because of the increased demand for glucose in a baby whose reserves may already be running low. Therefore, in severe cases or in babies who weigh less than expected for their gestational age (who may have less BAT), regular blood glucose monitoring and appropriate management are essential to maintain adequate levels of circulating glucose.

Point of note

If a baby has been warmed after becoming mildly hypothermic, their ability to maintain their temperature without the need of a heat source or extra clothing needs to be assessed before they are discharged home. An inability to maintain a normal core body temperature can indicate an underlying morbidity. It should also be noted that a baby may exhibit cutis marmorata (a mottling of the skin, often in the lower extremities), which is a vascular response in a baby who is re-warming after having been cold for a period of time, thus the question needs to be asked: why did they become cold in the first place? However, if this condition persists further investigation is required, as it may indicate poor perfusion as the result of developing sepsis, or it can be associated with trisomy 21, Edwards' (trisomy 18) and Cornelia de Lange syndromes.

13 Resuscitation of the newborn

Figure 13.1 Algorithm for newborn life support.
Source: Resuscitation Council UK (2021)/Resuscitation Council UK.

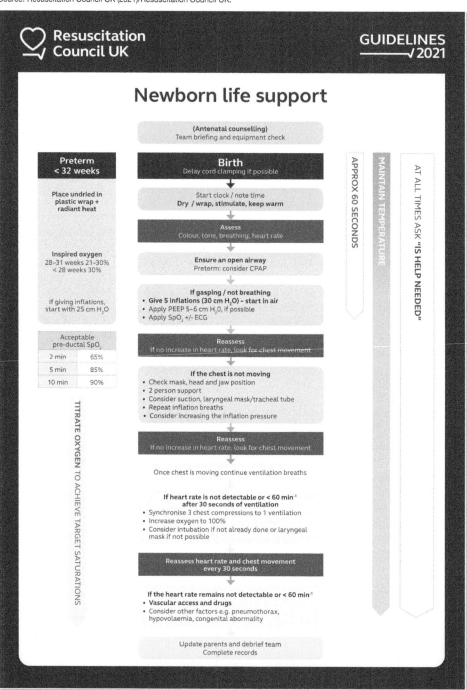

Physical Examination of the Newborn at a Glance, Second Edition. Dr Lyn Dolby and Denise (Dee) Campbell.
© 2025 John Wiley & Sons Ltd. Published 2025 by John Wiley & Sons Ltd.

Figure 13.2 (a–c) The neutral head position – essential for neonatal resuscitation.
Source: Lissauer et al. (2020)/John Wiley & Sons.

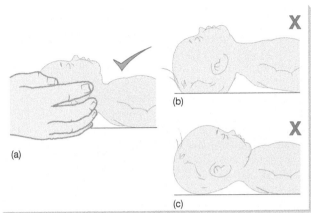

Figure 13.3 Sites for chest compression.
Source: Lissauer et al. (2020)/John Wiley & Sons.

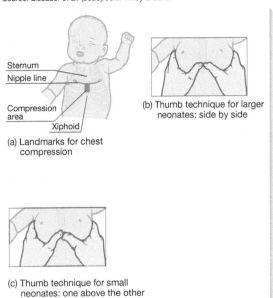

Figure 13.4 Algorithm for advanced newborn life support.
Source: Resuscitation Council UK (2021)/Resuscitation Council UK.

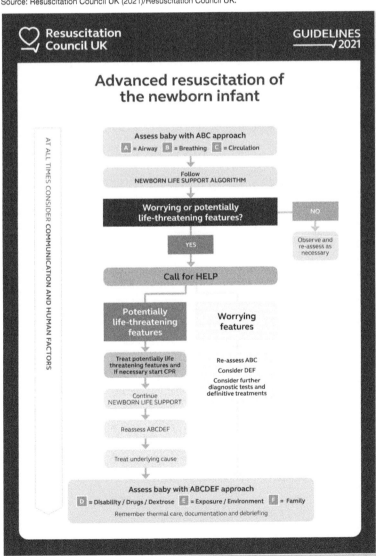

Resuscitation (Resuscitation Council UK et al., 2021b)

The practitioner could be called on to assist with any newborn resuscitation or have an infant collapse during the examination. Competence in resuscitation is essential.

Predisposing factors

Antenatal

- **Fetal**: growth restriction, prematurity, abnormality, multiple pregnancy, oligo- or poly-hydramnios.
- **Maternal**: infection, gestational diabetes, pregnancy-induced hypertension, pre-eclampsia, obesity, short stature, pre-term lack of steroids.

Intrapartum

- Evidence of fetal compromise (electrocardiogram [ECG], fetal blood sample, meconium-stained amniotic fluid).
- Breech vaginal delivery.
- Instrumental delivery (forceps or vacuum extraction).
- Significant bleeding.
- Caesarian section before 39 weeks or as an emergency.
- General anaesthetic.

Post-natal

- **Acute hypoxic incident**: airway obstruction, vaso-vagal attack, unclamped cord.
- **Chronic hypoxia**: hypothermia, pneumothorax, sepsis, abnormality, hypoglycaemia, metabolic disorder, heart disease.

Physiology

It is rare for the neonate to suffer a primary cardiac arrest without heart disease or congenital cardiac malformations. Most commonly a primary respiratory arrest occurs linked to hypoxia. The initial adaptive response is an increased respiratory effort – failure results in *primary apnoea*. Primitive respiratory centres then stimulate *agonal gasping* efforts in a final attempt to inflate the lungs before *terminal apnoea* follows. Increasing levels of lactic acid affect cardiac function, causing bradycardia to worsen until the heart stops. Commence life support if adequate, regular breathing has not established or if the heart rate (HR) is <100 beats/min.

Management (Figure 13.1) (Resuscitation Council UK, 2021; Resuscitation Council et al., 2021b)

The risk factors should be identified and the area for resuscitation prepared in advance. A warm, well-illuminated, flat surface is required (a resuscitaire provides a clock, oxygen, suction, heat, and pulse oximeter). The equipment is checked, the parents made aware (and consenting), and a paediatric team is available for support. If possible, the umbilical cord is not clamped for 60 seconds but, if it is clamped, cord milking is an option when the neonate is >34 weeks or >2 kg weight.

- Note the times (start the clock at birth).
- Assess breathing, HR, tone (and colour) every 30 seconds throughout – use a stethoscope and saturation monitoring.
- Keep the newborn warm and dry – hypothermia increases hypoglycaemia and acidosis. At birth, dry with a warm towel; replace this with a second warm, dry one (this also provides stimulation). Maintain newborn temperature between 36.5 and 37.5 °C – a hat/warm towel can assist in temperature control.
- Position the neonate with the chest clear to visualise their response to resuscitation.

Airway management: newborn not breathing

- Head in *neutral position* (Figure 13.2) – consider using a towel beneath the shoulders.
- Check *airway patency* – any suction must be 'direct vision' but is not required unless meconium, vernix or blood is seen obstructing the airway. Laryngoscopy is not recommended in the presence of meconium.
- Apply the correct-sized *mask*.
- Give *five inflation breaths* at 30 cm H_2O pressure (25 cm H_2O if the neonate is <32 weeks) for up to 2–3 seconds. The bag, valve, mask system uses air, mixed with oxygen only if SpO_2 levels require it in a term baby. Between 37 and 28 weeks pre-term the oxygen level is increased gradually up to 30%. Observe for chest movement – if it is not seen, reassess and follow the guidelines for absence of chest expansion in the next section. Then repeat the *inflation breaths*. When the airway is patent but inflation breaths are ineffective, increase the inflation pressure.
- Progress to *ventilation breaths* once chest expansion is seen – a rate of 30 breaths per min with 1 sec inflation time.
- *Stop* ventilation when HR>100 beats/min and breathing spontaneous.
- Monitor throughout with *pulse oximeter* on the right side – until acceptable HR and SpO_2 levels are reached (Figure 13.1).

Airway manoeuvres for absence of chest expansion

- Re-check the head is in a neutral position (Figure 13.2).
- Chin support – to prevent head flexion.
- Jaw forward (jaw lift) – if newborn tone is poor.
- Two-person airway control – one holds head and mask using jaw forward technique, the second operates the T-piece or bag.
- Guedel airway – to prevent tongue or soft tissue obstruction.
- Suction – laryngoscope (direct vision), paediatric Yankauer sucker.
- Laryngeal mask.
- Intubation.

Cardiac compressions: if HR <60 beats/min or absent after 30 seconds of ventilation

- Must be effective ventilation for cardiac compression to work. Add/increase to 100% oxygen.
- *Encircle chest* using two-hands technique (Figure 13.3).
- Apply *pressure* to lower third of sternum, avoiding the ziphoid process (Figure 13.3).
- *Depress* by one-third of the chest's AP diameter.
- Allow full *expansion* of the chest between compressions so the heart refills.
- The rate is 3 : 1 *cardiac compressions* to *ventilation breaths*, therefore 30 breaths and 90 compressions per minute.
- Use an ECG to continuously record HR (when available).
- *Stop* compressions when HR>60 beats/min.
- Consider *venous access and drugs* if HR<60 beats/min or not improving.

Drugs (S A D): if no response seen despite effective ventilation and cardiac compressions

• **S**odium bicarbonate – 4.2% solution. Dose 2–4 mL/kg^{-1} intravenous (IV).

• **A**drenaline (epinephrine) 1 : 10,000 solution. Dose 0.2 mL/kg^{-1} IV or intraosseous (IO), repeated every 3–5 min as required.

• **D**extrose/glucose 10%. Dose 250 mg/kg^{-1} bolus dose IV.

• Volume expander (if needed) – O Rh –ve blood or crystalloid as a bolus dose of 10 mL kg IV given over 10–20 s.

Stopping resuscitation

Ideally this will be when HR>100 beats/min and spontaneous breathing is present. In the unresponsive newborn, it will be when HR is not present or no longer present after 20 min of active resuscitation, when all reversible problems have been excluded. The Advanced Resuscitation Algorithm (Resuscitation Council UK et al., 2021a) will have been instigated if worrying/life threatening features were present (Figure 13.4).

14 Neonatal hypoglycaemia

Figure 14.1 Glucose metabolism.

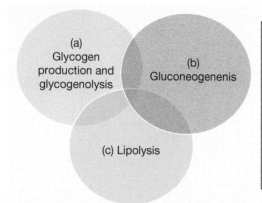

(a) Occurs mainly in the liver and muscles, but liver glycogen must be available (in fetus excess maternal glucose supplies are stored as glycogen in the liver)

(b) Requires substrates–amino acids, (particularly) alanine, lactate, pyruvate and glycerol

(c) Glycerol is metabolised from adipose tissue to be directly used in gluconeogenesis in the neonate. Lipolysis releases fatty acids and triglycerides that are metabolised to ketonebodies → used directly in energy production → brain. Infant feeding (particularly breast milk) stimulates ketone body production

Table 14.1 Causes of hypoglycaemia.

Decreased levels of substrate	Premature babies Multiple births Fetal growth restriction (see summary of recommendations for full criteria in British Association of Perinatal Medicine, 2024)
Increased glucose requirements	Hyperinsulinaemia Baby of a mother with diabetes Rhesus isoimmunisation Hypertrophy of the pancreas (nesidioblastosis) Islet cell tumour Beckwith–Wiedemann syndrome Polycythaemia
Inability to utilise glucose	Glycogen storage disease Galactosaemia Fructose intolerance Inborn errors of metabolism
Miscellaneous and/ or accessory to	Birth asphyxia Endocrine deficiencies (e.g. congenial adrenal hyperplasia) Hypopituitarism

Table 14.2 Risk factors that instigate immediate investigation and management.

Babies with a history of predisposing factors	Babies with one or more of the following conditions or clinical signs
Babies of mothers with diabetes	Perinatal acidosis (cord arterial or infant pH <7.1 and base deficit >8 mmol [moderate] and >12 mmol [severe] metabolic acidosis) Hypothermia (<36.5 °C)
Babies whose mothers have been prescribed beta-blockers	Suspected or confirmed early-onset sepsis Cyanosis Apnoea Seizures
Babies with intrauterine growth restriction with a birth weight ≤2nd centile and term babies who have a 'clinically wasted' appearance, babies who are premature or part of a multiple birth N.B. The parameters **must** be measured using a sex-specific centile chart	Hypotonia Lethargy Altered level of consciousness High-pitched cry

Table 14.3 Operational thresholds for management.

A value <1.0 mmol/L at any time
A single value <2.5 mmol/L in a neonate with abnormal clinical signs
More than two measurements <2.0 mmol/L in a baby with a risk factor for impaired metabolic adaptation and hypoglycaemia but without abnormal clinical signs

A transient rise in fetal glucose concentrations from glycogenolysis and gluconeogenesis occurs close to the baby's birth. At birth the placental connection is lost, a rapid decline in neonatal glucose levels then follows, reaching a nadir at 1–2 hours of age. Without the steady maternal supply of glucose via the placenta, a strong ketogenic response is instigated through the processes involved in glucose metabolism (Figure 14.1). As a result, the blood glucose concentration rises again to a level similar to that in late fetal gestation at approximately 2–4 hours post birth. By 3–4 days post birth, the blood glucose level will have reached the adult level. However, if any part of the process of glucose metabolism is disrupted, hypoglycaemia can rapidly develop (see Table 14.1 for causes of neonatal hypoglycaemia).

Hypoglycaemia occurs when the blood sugar concentration drops below a pre-determined level, causing the appearance of clinical symptoms. This event occurs in about 1–3 out of every 1000 births. However, there has been much discussion relating to how low the level of blood glucose can fall in relation to the baby's age before physiological compromise and long-term issues develop (Hay, 2022; Roeper et al., 2023).

Glucose and oxygen are the main sources of fuel utilised by the human brain. Without adequate blood sugar levels (or oxygen), the brain's ability to function is initially impaired. As the state of hypoglycaemia continues or becomes severe, there is an ever-increasing likelihood of seizures, permanent injury to the brain and long-term neurodevelopmental impairment. Therefore, it is important for practitioners to appreciate both national and local guidelines in order to be able to detect those babies who may have a predisposition to becoming hypoglycaemic as well as to understand the clinical signs that may appear with a fall in glucose levels.

Predisposing factors

Immediate investigation and management should be instigated in babies who have known predisposing risk factors and/or in those who demonstrate one or more clinical signs (Table 14.2). However, it should be noted that 'jitteriness' is common in neonates and is not in itself an indication to measure blood glucose (jitteriness is witnessed as excessive repetitive movements of one or more limbs that are unprovoked and not in response to a stimulus). It should also be remembered that neonates do not display the usual autonomic nervous system response seen in adults, for example sweating and pallor. The British Association of Perinatal Medicine (BAPM) guidance (2024) also states that babies who are large for their gestational age do not require routine screening unless there is evidence of maternal diabetes or the presence of dysmorphic features associated with Beckwith–Wiedemann syndrome. However, as with any baby, hypoglycaemia can be asymptomatic in its presentation. An apparently 'normal' baby may have a latent condition – such as infection – that may influence their requirement for energy and affect levels of circulating glucose. Therefore, any increase or decrease in temperature or abnormal feeding behaviour (e.g. not suckling effectively or waking for feeds, unsettled or demanding frequent feeds) should prompt further assessment and investigation of blood glucose levels. Hay (2022) reiterates the difficulty with clinically assessing for asymptomatic hypoglycaemia and the debate relating to blood glucose levels in the newborn and their significance in terms of health of the child in later years.

BAPM (2024) highlights the importance of assessing all babies at birth for risk of hypoglycaemia. For those with risk factors, the BAPM Newborn Early Warning Trigger and Track (NEWTT2) chart should be consulted, as it gives a visual assessment of the baby's condition and is a useful aid in the detection of hypoglycaemia. The NEWTT2 chart can be accessed at https://www.bapm.org/pages/newtt-2.

Neonatal blood glucose assessment

Diagnosis and treatment of neonatal hypoglycaemia require accurate measurement of blood glucose levels. Significant inaccuracy can occur with current cot-side technology, particularly within the range of 0–2.0 mmol/L. Even with equipment that has been validated for neonatal use, there is a possible error of ±0.5 mmol/L for values <5.5 mmol/L.

It is recommended (BAPM, 2024) that blood gas analysers as used in neonatal units, if calibrated and utilised by trained practitioners, can provide accurate results at low blood glucose levels. It is important to note that they can provide a glucose level report without providing results that have not been clinically requested. See Table 14.3 for BAPM guidance (2024) relating to blood glucose thresholds requiring management.

Training

Roeper et al. (2023) reiterate the past work of Hawdon et al. (2017) in that there is still a need for the provision of adequate training for all those involved in neonatal care. The BAPM guidance (2024) promotes this requirement and also that training should include the need to avoid separating mothers and babies, and ultimately reduce unnecessary investigations in those babies not at risk and who do not demonstrate clinical signs. BAPM also advocate that maternity units adopt the UNICEF UK Baby Friendly standards tool (https://www.unicef.org.uk/babyfriendly) to assist in training and assessment of feeding during the first week of life. The tool should help focus the attention of healthcare workers on the ability of the baby to feed, promote breastfeeding support and enable recognition of poor feeding that may contribute to hypoglycaemia. Additionally, the BAPM provides flowcharts to aid in the management of those babies who are at risk of hypoglycaemia, those who are found to have low blood sugar levels and term newborns who are reluctant feeders but otherwise 'healthy'.

15 Physiological jaundice

Figure 15.1 The process of bilirubin metabolism.

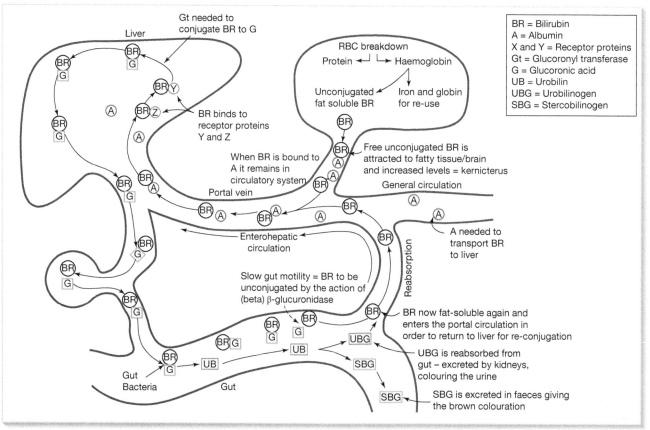

Table 15.1 Factors that adversely affect bilirubin metabolism.

Site	Effect on bilirubin metabolism
Spleen	Increased haemolysis leads to excessive bilirubin levels
General circulation/ portal vein	Shortage of plasma albumin to bind with unconjugated fat-soluble bilirubin allows it to exit the circulatory system where, because of its attraction to fatty tissue/brain, high levels can cause kernicterus
Liver	Hypoxia and hypoglycaemia reduce the level of metabolism as both O_2 and glucose are necessary for the process to work. Glucose is the raw material used for the production of glucuronic acid
Liver → gall bladder	Biliary obstruction leads to obstructive jaundice Low levels of enteric bacteria
Gut	Slow gut mobility leads to bilirubin becoming unconjugated again because of the action of beta-glucuronidase

Physical Examination of the Newborn at a Glance, Second Edition. Dr Lyn Dolby and Denise (Dee) Campbell.
© 2025 John Wiley & Sons Ltd. Published 2025 by John Wiley & Sons Ltd.

Table 15.2 Predisposing factors that require extra vigilance.

Bruises or trauma at delivery	Can exacerbate jaundice due to increased breakdown of red blood cells
Previous sibling with jaundice in neonatal period requiring phototherapy	Extra and early assessment is required – use of transcutaneous bilirubin measurement or serum bilirubin
Ethnicity	Highly pigmented babies have a higher risk of jaundice, e.g. Arabian ethnic background equals a higher risk of glucose-6-phosphate dehydrogenase deficiency (G6PD)
Poor feeders	Lower fluid intake and slower evacuation of the bowel can reduce capability to excrete bilirubin from the body
Growth restricted, small for dates babies	Can have reduced ability to metabolise bilirubin particularly as often there is a higher level of organ immaturity
Exclusively breastfed	Does not occur in all exclusively breastfed babies
Rhesus-negative mother	Antibody reports should be investigated and baby's status assessed more frequently
Maternal infection/neonatal infection	The physiological response to infection can reduce the ability of the body to metabolise bilirubin efficiently

Source: Adapted from NICE (2023a).

Table 15.3 Management – positive actions and negative signs.

Positive actions	Negative signs
Skin to skin continues to aid natural biome = supportive function Early, frequent feeds Observe quality of feed and willingness of baby to suckle and state of alertness/general well-being Frequent feeds for those babies who are small for their gestational age even if they need to be woken for feeds (e.g. 3 hourly) Give expressed breastmilk if necessary Supplementation with artificial formula milk – only if baby is unable to suckle	Depth of colour (yellow) is becoming more marked/widespread Baby is lethargic, sleepy, difficult to rouse Passage of 'pale' stools Baby demonstrates decreased muscle tone, high-pitched cry or increasing development of 'unusual' movement

Note: Placing baby in sunlight (even indirectly/filtered) can cause dehydration from overheating and sunburn as their skin layers are thinner than those of an adult, plus there is less protective melanin (Nutfilloyevna and Shokir qizi, 2024).

Physiological jaundice is the deposition of bilirubin (a weak, fat-soluble, yellow-pigmented acid) in the newborn skin, sclera and mucous membranes (NICE, 2023a). Bilirubin is the by-product of bilirubin metabolism that marks the end of the lifespan of a red blood cell (RBC). This process of RBC destruction occurs in the reticuloendothelial system (liver, spleen and macrophages). The characteristic yellow discolouration of the skin becomes visible as excess bilirubin levels rise and may be a result of physiological or pathological conditions or breastmilk jaundice.

Entry of unconjugated bilirubin into the brain (causing the characteristic yellow staining of the tissue) can cause both short- and long-term neurological dysfunction (bilirubin encephalopathy). The clinical features associated with acute or chronic bilirubin encephalopathy are collectively termed kernicterus. The risk of kernicterus increases in babies with extremely high bilirubin levels. Kernicterus is also known to occur at lower levels of bilirubin in term babies who have predisposing risk factors and in those babies who are pre-term.

Bilirubin metabolism

The process of bilirubin metabolism is shown in Figure 15.1, demonstrating the factors on which the process is dependent to enable unconjugated (free) bilirubin to become conjugated (bound) and safely excreted from the neonate via the urine and faeces. However, the neonatal liver is still maturing and the mechanism of bilirubin metabolism depends on a healthy infant who is feeding adequately. Factors that can adversely affect bilirubin metabolism are highlighted in Table 15.1.

In the United Kingdom, physiological jaundice occurs in approximately 50% of term babies each year. A much higher proportion of pre-term babies (80%) will become jaundiced as a result of organ immaturity and accompanying disorders of prematurity.

During fetal life, the placenta and maternal liver manage fetal RBC breakdown. Although the fetus can conjugate small quantities of bilirubin, the fetal liver is relatively inactive, taking over bilirubin metabolism only at birth. The enzyme beta-glucuronidase, present in the fetus's small-bowel luminal brush border, is released into the intestinal lumen, where it deconjugates bilirubin glucuronide. Free (unconjugated) bilirubin is then re-absorbed from the gastrointestinal tract and re-enters the fetal circulation. Fetal bilirubin is cleared from the circulation by placental transfer into the mother's plasma following a concentration gradient. The maternal liver then takes on the process of bilirubin metabolism by conjugating and excreting the fetal bilirubin until this placental connection is terminated at birth.

The neonatal liver continues to conjugate and excrete bilirubin into bile so it can be eliminated in the stool. However, because of the lack of intestinal bacteria for oxidising bilirubin to urobilinogen in the gut, the unaltered bilirubin remains in the stool, giving the typical bright yellow colour. In addition, the neonatal gastrointestinal tract (like that of the fetus) contains beta-glucuronidase, which deconjugates some of the bilirubin. When the neonate feeds, the gastro-colic reflex is stimulated, causing bilirubin to be excreted via the stools before most of it can be deconjugated and reabsorbed. Nevertheless, in some neonates, particularly those who are not feeding as well or as frequently as would be expected, lack of bowel evacuation leads to the unconjugated bilirubin being re-absorbed and returned to the circulation from the intestinal lumen (entero-hepatic circulation of bilirubin), contributing to physiological hyperbilirubinaemia and jaundice.

Incidence and risk factors

Predisposing risk factors for babies are outlined in Table 15.2. Ethnicity is also a factor, depending on place of birth, as those with ethnic routes from Asia or South America (excluding those not born in their home country) would appear to have a greater propensity towards jaundice than those with European and African ancestry. Every time a practitioner examines a baby who has a higher level of pigmentation (including Mediterranean heritage) it is important to conduct a physical assessment for jaundice, as a visual assessment alone will not identify jaundice. A comprehensive demonstration of how this should be performed is available at https://www.youtube.com/watch?v=sQlSMYjJ0OY.

Presentation and management

Physiological jaundice usually appears around day 3–4 and then fades over the next 10 days. Stools and urine should be of a normal colour and the baby is seen to feed as expected for their gestation and post-birth age while demonstrating normal posture/movement and responsiveness. A healthy asymptomatic neonate does not usually require treatment. It is also important to consider parental skin colour and observe the baby in good natural light, as yellow–green clothing, bedding and window coverings can make a baby appear jaundiced even when they are not.

Neonatal jaundice follows a cephalopedal colour progression (head, upper torso, lower torso, arms/legs, hands and feet). A transcutaneous bilirubinometer (TcB) can be used to measure the bilirubin level in babies whose gestational age is ≥35 weeks and who are over 24 hours of age. If a TcB is unavailable or the measurement indicates a bilirubin level >250 µmmol/L (lower limits may apply locally), a total serum bilirubin (TSB) test should be carried out to check the result. The neonate must be referred to the neonatologist for decisions regarding treatment and further investigation as to cause. The TSB result must be recorded on a TSB chart that is appropriate for the gestational age of the neonate. However, in the event of jaundice occurring in the first 24–48 hours of life, a TSB should be the first course of action.

Positive actions and negative signs

Parents need to be aware of the positive actions they can take to assist the physiological process of bilirubin metabolism, as well as the possible negative changes to observe in their baby's general health that may indicate the level of jaundice is increasing as a result of pathological causes (Table 15.3). They need to know how to contact their healthcare professional in the event of any concern or negative changes in their baby's behaviour or colour, so that urgent referral for assessment and/or treatment can be expedited.

Urgent referral to the paediatric team for assessment and TSB must always occur in the event of jaundice developing within 24 hours of birth and also if at any time a neonate appears to be significantly jaundiced and lethargic or dehydrated. The same action applies in the case of jaundice developing after 7 days or remaining after 14 days when causation has not been identified in an otherwise well (asymptomatic) baby.

Jaundice associated with breastfeeding

In 15% of cases, where jaundice becomes prolonged (beyond two weeks of age) it can be associated with breastfeeding unless the baby is found to have another condition. Glucoronyl transferase is inhibited by hormones in breastmilk and further breastmilk hormones can cause conjugated bilirubin to revert to an unconjugated state. Slow bacterial colonisation of the gut due to relatively low volumes of milk that the baby imbibes during the first three days exacerbates this process. If earlier initiation of breastfeeding has been problematic, extra support will prove beneficial and confidence building. However, if the baby appears well and is feeding, even if having to be woken to do so, parents should be reassured and encouraged to continue breastfeeding and feed their baby frequently.

Professional note: The present provision of postnatal visiting does not allow for adequate assessment for jaundice, particularly in highly pigmented babies. As students and practitioners in midwifery you are no doubt well aware that this is **not** the only aspect of midwifery care that as professionals we may be judged on in terms of how a practitioner exercises their role and responsibility in a professional manner within the remit of the leadership section of 'The Code' (NMC, 2018). Review your NHS Trust's processes and reflect on how postnatal visiting is managed and whether conditions are recognised in a timely manner within present service provisions, in particular for those more at risk or vulnerable. If at times phone calls are used, reflect on how this links with your understanding of 'comprehensive assessment', professional autonomy and leadership.

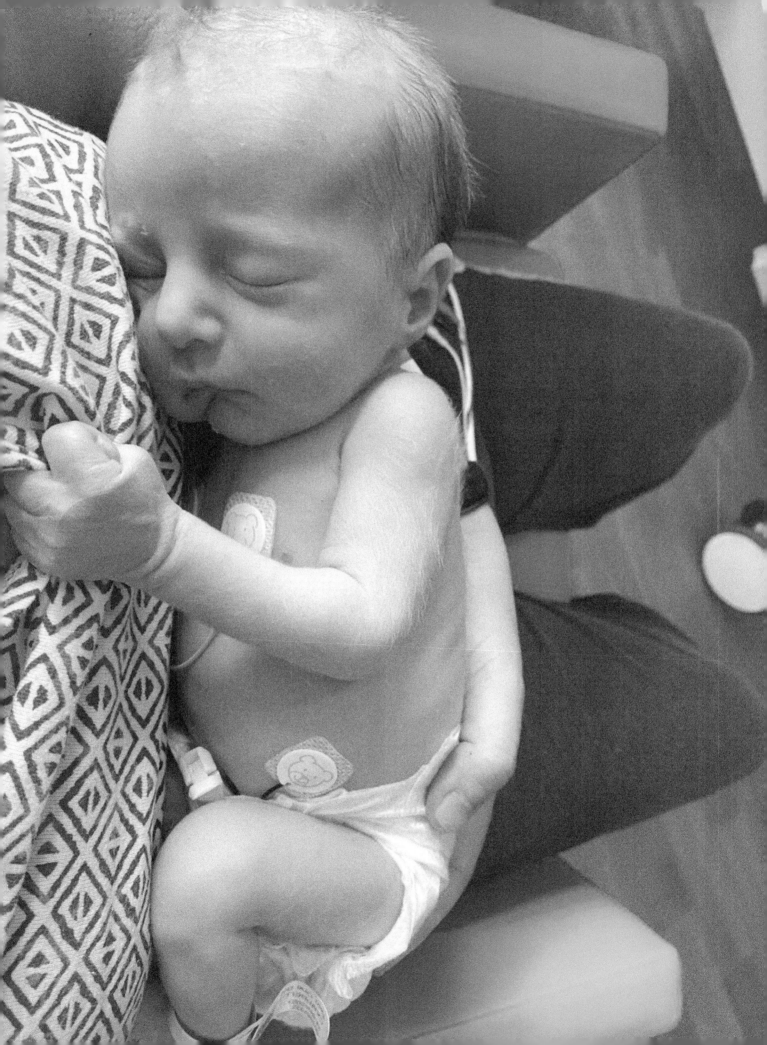

Pathological jaundice

Table 16.1 Factors that adversely affect bilirubin metabolism.

Factor	Effect
Increased haemolysis	Can lead to excessive bilirubin levels – possible causes include haemolytic disease of the newborn and maternal drug therapy (e.g. sulphonamides)
Shortage of albumin	Albumin is needed to bind with unconjugated fat-soluble bilirubin; shortage may be caused by low serum albumin levels, asphyxia, acidosis, infection, hypoglycaemia and prematurity Particular drugs (e.g. sulphonamides and sodium benzoate) can also bind with albumin and compete with bilirubin
Hypoxia and hypoglycaemia	Both reduce the level of metabolism as both O_2 and glucose are necessary for the process to work. Glucose is the raw material used for the production of glucuronic acid
Low levels of gut bacteria and reduced peristalsis	Low levels of gut bacteria are normal at birth. Feeding encourages the population of normal fauna and flora in the neonatal gut and stimulates peristalsis. Slow or delayed initiation of feeding provides the circumstances that allow conjugated bilirubin to deconjugate (via action of beta-glucuronidase) and re-enter the hepatic circulation

Table 16.3 Possible causes of unconjugated and conjugated jaundice.

Unconjugated jaundice (often referred to as 'indirect', which circulates bound bilirubin to albumin but some remains free and can be deposited in the brain tissue)	
Day 1	Haemolytic disease of the newborn
Days 2–5	Haemolytic disease of the newborn; jaundice of prematurity; sepsis; extravascular blood; spherocytosis; polycythaemia and glucose-6-phosphate dehydrogenase deficiency (G6PD)
Days 5–10	Sepsis; galactosaemia and hypothyroidism
Day 10+	Sepsis, urinary tract infection and breastmilk jaundice
Conjugated jaundice (this form has been metabolised in the liver, often referred to as 'direct', and is excreted via the faeces)	
Days 1–10	Neonatal hepatitis; rubella; cytomegalovirus (CMV) and syphilis
Day 10+	*Biliary obstruction* causes obstructive jaundice, whereby the flow of bile is prevented from flowing into the intestine, allowing a quantity of bilirubin to escape back into the bloodstream

Table 16.2 Serious outcomes of untreated high serum bilirubin levels.

Bilirubin encephalopathy	A condition that is reversible
Brain damage	Irreversible as it results in severe learning difficulties
Kernicterus	A rare but often fatal condition in which toxic levels of unconjugated bilirubin migrate to fatty tissue of the central nervous system causing irreversible damage to the basal ganglia of the brain **Note**: Kernicterus is nearly always preventable except in very sick or premature babies

Table 16.4 Urgent referral for admission for neonatal assessment.

Time period	Criteria for referral/admission
Within 2 hours	Jaundice in the first 24 hours of life
Within 6 hours	Jaundice first appears at more than 7 days of age Neonate is unwell (e.g. lethargy, fever, vomiting, irritability) Gestational age <35 weeks Prolonged jaundice: • Gestational age <37 weeks + jaundice for >21 days • Gestational age ≥37 weeks + jaundice for >14 days Poor feeding and/or concerns regarding weight, particularly if breastfed Pale stools and dark urine

Table 16.5 Further investigations.

Investigation	Finding	Possible cause
Full blood count and blood film	↑ or ↓ white blood cell count or thrombocytopenia	Sepsis
	Haematocrit <45%	Haemolytic anaemia
	↑ Reticulocyte count	Haemolysis
Blood group and rhesus factor (mother and baby)	Maternal blood group O/ baby blood group A or B	ABO incompatibility
	Mother rhesus negative/ baby rhesus positive	Rhesus isoimmunisation
Liver function tests	Increased liver enzymes	Congenital infection
Blood G6PD levels	Presence of G6PD – usually occurs in relation to ethnicity and sex	

G6PD, glucose-6-phosphate dehydrogenase deficiency.

Physical Examination of the Newborn at a Glance, Second Edition. Dr Lyn Dolby and Denise (Dee) Campbell.
© 2025 John Wiley & Sons Ltd. Published 2025 by John Wiley & Sons Ltd.

As can be seen in Chapter 15, the process of bilirubin metabolism is complex and dependent on a number of factors to enable unconjugated ('indirect') bilirubin to become conjugated ('direct') and sent to the gut to be excreted via the faeces. The factors that can adversely affect bilirubin metabolism are highlighted in Table 16.1, but physiological jaundice is not the result of an underlying pathological condition. Professional vigilance in observing for risk factors within the maternal and neonatal documentation (see Chapter 15, Table 15.2) and continual assessment of the baby's colour and well-being are vital for early detection. This is particularly important in the event that physiological and pathological jaundice occur together, for example prolonged jaundice may include breastfeeding jaundice, a normally occurring physiological condition that could mask something more serious such as biliary atresia. The aim in 'pathological' jaundice is not only to prevent the level of bilirubin from rising further, but also to diagnose and treat the underlying cause(s) in order to prevent ongoing hyperbilirubinaemia.

The concern with hyperbilirubinaemia is that it has a high affinity to fatty tissue such as the brain. Elevated levels of unconjugated bilirubin deposited in the neurons of the brain are neurotoxic and can cause acute or chronic encephalopathy. Kernicterus, or bilirubin encephalopathy, is a condition caused by bilirubin toxicity to the basal ganglia and various brainstem nuclei, the outcomes of which are highlighted in Table 16.2. Therefore, an awareness of the risk factors that are associated with pathological jaundice is paramount.

Pathological risk factors

The causes of unconjugated and conjugated jaundice can be seen in Table 16.3. Table 16.4 indicates the usual neonatal age at which a specific factor may appear or be detected. The factors that can cause pathological jaundice include those that directly cause haemolysis of the red blood cells (e.g. rhesus or ABO incompatibility); excessive bruising and extravascular blood leakage; sepsis; metabolic disorders (e.g. galactosaemia, hereditary fructose intolerance, hypothyroidism, alpha-1 antitrypsin deficiency); Gilbert's syndrome and Crigler–Najjar syndrome (which although rare are caused by liver enzyme anomalies); glucose-6-phosphate dehydrogenase (G6PD) deficiency (a familial enzyme deficiency most common in Mediterranean, Middle Eastern, South-East Asian and African populations); and malformation or congenital obstruction of the biliary system such as biliary atresia (conjugated hyperbilirubinaemia arising from obstructive jaundice).

Assessment

Assessment during the first 48 hours is essential if there is a history of possible risk factors. The parents should be asked whether the baby's siblings or close family relatives experienced neonatal jaundice that required phototherapy or exchange blood transfusion. Investigate the ability of the baby to feed or if difficult to arouse, the daily number of wet and dirty nappies and the colour of urine and stools. Check for signs of illness or fever, evidence of new or increased bleeding or bruising.

Always assess the baby's colour in bright natural light at every contact opportunity within the first 72 hours of birth (NICE, 2023a). Evaluate the colour of the whole body, noting any colour change in the sclerae, gums or palate or when pressing lightly on the nose or chest. See Chapter 15 for a link relating to assessment of babies with darker skin tones. However, do not rely on visual inspection alone but measure the bilirubin level with appropriate equipment. Adverse findings should instigate direct, urgent referral to a neonatologist, who should also be informed of the result of a TcB measurement if performed (NICE, 2023a).

Bilirubin measurement: when to record

- **First 24 hours or gestational age <35 weeks:** Use serum bilirubin (SBR) measurement within 2 hours and continue to measure SBR every 6 hours until the level is both below the treatment threshold and stable or falling. Bilirubin levels should be interpreted according to the baby's postnatal age in hours by plotting the results on an appropriate threshold graph (see NICE, 2023a, and the link at the end of the chapter).
- **≥24 hours post birth:** Measure and record bilirubin level urgently (within 6 hours) in all babies with suspected or obvious jaundice and refer urgently if necessary.

Bilirubin measurement: equipment

- **SBR measurement:** Babies in first 24 hours of life or whose gestational age is <35 weeks.
- **Transcutaneous bilirubinometer (TcB):** For babies who are ≥35 weeks and over 24 hours of age, use a TcB (if not available use SBR). If TcB indicates a bilirubin level >250 μmol/L, measure SBR. Use SBR if bilirubin levels are at or above the relevant treatment thresholds for the baby's age and for all subsequent measurements.

Note: There is ongoing research in relation to correct SBR values between 35 and 40 weeks' gestation that may change practices in the future.

Further investigations

In order to detect underlying causes, further investigations such as those in Table 16.5 should be conducted. Although investigations also include umbilical cord blood direct antiglobulin test (DAT) and Coombs' test, this should only be used to diagnose ABO or rhesus isoimmunisation and not to predict significant hyperbilirubinaemia (NICE, 2023a). Microbiological cultures in relation to blood, urine and cerebrospinal fluid may also be investigated if infection is suspected but the source of the infection is unclear.

Treatment of choice

Treatment depends on the SBR level and/or cause of the jaundice. Therefore, appropriate treatment will be given to a baby with an underlying illness such as an infection. Phototherapy will be used if the SBR is at or above the treatment threshold in order to assist the conversion of unconjugated bilirubin into products that can be more easily excreted from the body via the stools and urine. An exchange transfusion is required in a baby with signs of bilirubin encephalopathy and who may be at risk of kernicterus or if the baby is not responding to phototherapy. If the underlying cause for jaundice is a condition such as biliary atresia, then early admission for surgery will be the appropriate treatment of choice.

Parental support

Parents require a great deal of support from the moment the baby becomes visibly jaundiced or sleepy and reluctant to feed until the jaundice is resolved and any underlying cause treated. For some parents this latter point may not be resolved easily or without further anxiety (e.g. G6PD). Discussion with parents needs to be clear, concise and in a language and terminology that they can understand. In some cases, directing them to groups or associations in relation to specific conditions will assist in the ongoing support they may need.

Jaundice in the newborn should never be underestimated and the NICE clinical guideline will help you be further informed: https://www.nice.org.uk/guidance/cg98.

17 Metabolic disorders

Figure 17.1 Early signs and symptoms of metabolic disorder, showing deterioration pattern if untreated (some or all of the features may present).

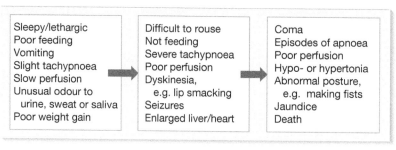

Sleepy/lethargic
Poor feeding
Vomiting
Slight tachypnoea
Slow perfusion
Unusual odour to
   urine, sweat or saliva
Poor weight gain
	Difficult to rouse
	Not feeding
	Severe tachypnoea
	Poor perfusion
	Dyskinesia,
	   e.g. lip smacking
	Seizures
	Enlarged liver/heart
		Coma
		Episodes of apnoea
		Poor perfusion
		Hypo- or hypertonia
		Abnormal posture,
		   e.g. making fists
		Jaundice
		Death

Figure 17.2 Flow chart for newborn blood-spot test screening. GP, general practitioner; HV, health visitor; MW, midwife; PCHR, personal child health record.

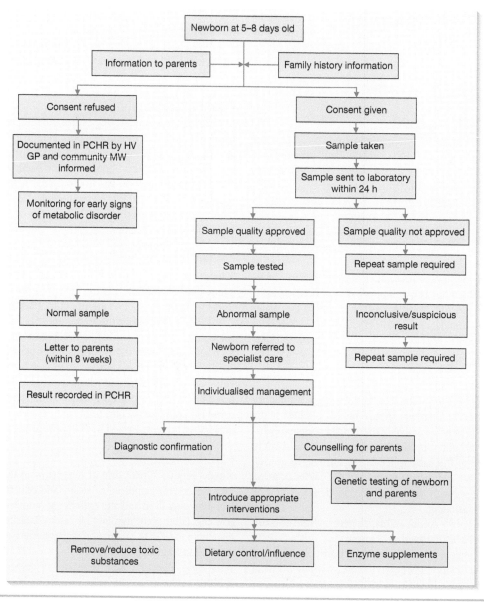

Physical Examination of the Newborn at a Glance, Second Edition. Dr Lyn Dolby and Denise (Dee) Campbell.
© 2025 John Wiley & Sons Ltd. Published 2025 by John Wiley & Sons Ltd.

Metabolic disorders

This chapter aims to increase understanding around metabolic disorders in the newborn. There are known to be hundreds of genetic metabolic disorders, which can result from even the most basic mutation of a gene. It will not be possible to cover them all, so the aim will be to raise awareness generally and to mention some of the most common disorders. The chapter should be read in conjunction with those on associated risk factors, hypo- and hyperglycaemia, genetics and inheritance.

What are metabolic disorders?

Metabolic disorders are a failure in the normal enzyme processes that break down and convert ingested food into essential proteins and amino acids, needed for normal body function. The result is either an excess or deficit of the end products of metabolism. Too much and the body has to store them in the liver, body fat or muscle, where excess levels can become toxic and damage cells. Too little and the specific cells cannot work normally, leading to failures in whole body systems.

Causes of metabolic disorders

In the majority of newborn cases a mutated gene is responsible. This is more commonly inherited, but can also occur for the first time with no family member affected. It is important to remember this and not to judge a newborn's parentage. A mutated gene can cause:
* A deficiency in an enzyme or compound required for metabolism – the most common cause of a metabolic disorder.
* A genetic disorder of (or damage to) any of the organs involved in metabolism, e.g. liver or pancreas.
* An abnormal chemical reaction occurring during metabolism.

It is also possible for a dietary vitamin or mineral deficiency, or excess, to cause a metabolic disorder. When breastfeeding or bottle feeding (using specially formulated artificial feeds), a problem of diet is rare in the newborn. It could occur in situations where inappropriate or incorrect artificial feeds are being given or when a breastfeeding mother has a severely deficient diet.

Types of congenital metabolic disorders

There are believed to be 800–1000 types of congenital metabolic disorders. The numbers and varieties make classification a challenge. Very simply they can be seen to align within four main categories:
* **Disorders of metabolism** – deficiency of the enzymes required for synthesis of:
  * Carbohydrates, e.g. diabetes, galactosemia.
  * Amino acids, e.g. phenylketonuria (PKU), maple syrup disease.
  * Metal, e.g. Wilson's disease.
  * Steroids, e.g. congenital adrenal hyperplasia.
  * Fatty acids, e.g. medium-chain acyl-coenzyme A dehydrogenase deficiency (MCADD).
* **Disorder of the urea cycle** – deficiency of one of six enzymes required for removal of waste products, e.g. carbamylphosphate synthetase 1.
* **Disorders of mitochondrial function** – dysfunction of cells converting foods into the energy they need, e.g. Kearns-Sayre syndrome.
* **Disorders specific to lysosomal or peroxisomal storage** – deficiency or absence of the enzymes that break down toxins within cell spaces, e.g. Zellweger syndrome, Gaucher disease, Tay-Sachs disease, cystic fibrosis.

Signs, symptoms and screening

These are dependent on the exact type of disorder, disease or syndrome. Presentation at birth can be as extreme as hydrops fetalis (Gaucher disease) or dysmorphic features (Zellweger syndrome). In most cases there will be no signs at birth, then a gradual onset of neurological symptoms, metabolic acidosis and/or hypoglycaemia. Progression may lead to cardiac disease, liver dysfunction, bone damage, central nervous system (CNS) damage and death.

Routine screening in the early newborn period is via the newborn blood-spot test, which can detect a number of disorders before significant symptoms or harm can occur (Figure 17.2). Detection otherwise may be due to raised concerns from family history or signs of early onset. A deterioration pattern often begins with a sleepy baby, feeding problems and failure to thrive (see Figure 17.1).

Principles of treatment

These conditions cannot be cured but instead must be managed to limit damaging side effects. The three main principles involved are:
* Alteration of the diet to remove (or prevent the introduction of) any foods that cannot be digested.
* Introduction of enzymes or supplements to correct imbalance.
* Treatment to remove or reduce any toxic substances.

Most common congenital metabolic disorders

All of the individual conditions are relatively rare but, since so many exist, the chance of a newborn baby having one of the disorders is increased. It is likely that all practitioners will come across a metabolic disorder at least once in their career. Those based in the community or involved in longer-term care will meet them more frequently. The more common ones are:
* **Congenital adrenal hyperplasia**: typically the adrenal glands produce insufficient cortisol and too many androgens, which may result in ambiguous genitalia.
* **Cystic fibrosis**: a recessive inherited disorder affecting the exocrine glands. Sodium and chlorine excess in cells cause dehydrated, thickened mucus secretions within the lung cells.
* **Diabetes mellitus**: may be type 1 (insulin dependent) or type 2 and results from genetic factors or uncontrolled maternal diabetes, including gestational forms.
* **Galactosemia**: inability to break down galactose to glucose.
* **Gaucher disease**: an excess of glucosylceramide; more severe forms affect the nervous system. The most common inherited genetic condition among Ashkenazi Jews.
* **Maple syrup disease**: inability to break down certain amino acids; severity ranges from mild to severe (when brain damage can occur). Named because of the sweet maple smell of the urine.
* **MCADD**: inability to break down medium-chain fatty acids into acetyl-CoA; symptoms include hypoglycaemia and sudden death.
* **PKU**: inability to break down phenylalanine, which builds up in the blood and brain.
* **Tay-Sachs disease**: gangliosides accumulate in the brain causing progressive damage from 7 months, death by 4 years.
* **Wilson's disease**: the body is unable to remove excess copper storage, mainly in the brain and liver.
* **Zellweger syndrome**: life-threatening, multi-system failure to break down toxins. Facial and skeletal dysmorphia often present.

18 Jitteriness, seizures and hypotonia

Table 18.1 Distinguishing jitteriness from convulsions (seizures).

	Jitteriness	Convulsions
Stimulus provoked	Yes	No
Predominant movement	Rapid, oscillatory	Clonic, tonic
Movements cease when limb is held	Yes	No
Conscious state	Awake or asleep	Altered
Eye deviation	No	Yes

Source: Sinha et al. (2018)/John Wiley & Sons.

Table 18.3 Causes of newborn hypotonia.

Paralytic	Non-paralytic
Spinal muscular atrophy (Werdnig-Hoffmann)	Birth asphyxia
Congenital muscular dystrophy	Down's syndrome
Congenital myopathy	Prader-Willi syndrome
Congenital myotonic dystrophy	Skeletal and connective tissue disorders
Myasthenia gravis	Drugs
Benign congenital hypotonia

Source: Sinha et al. (2018) / John Wiley & Sons.

Box 18.1   Signs of subtle neonatal seizures

- Staring, locked eye position
- Eyes contracted to one side
- Lip-smacking movements
- Sucking lower lip
- Sucking tongue
- Pedalling legs
- Swimming movements of upper and/or lower limbs
- Apnoea
- *Electroencephalogram (EEG) required to confirm seizure*

Box 18.2   Types of neonatal seizures

- **Subtle**: the most common type in the first six weeks of life (see Box 18.1).
- **Focal clonic**: repetitive, rhythmic jerking of a small area (tongue, face, diaphragm) or large area (limb, head). May start in one area then spread to opposite side or further within the same side.
- **Focal tonic**: continuous but short-lasting muscle contraction; symmetrical or asymmetrical. May include deviation of eyes. If generalised there may be extension of all extremities or upper flexion and lower extension.
- **Myoclonic**: non-repetitive, arrhythmic contraction, affecting a small area (e.g. finger) or whole body. May mimic Moro reflex.

These can also be:
- Multifocal.
- Generalised.

Source: Adapted from Krawiec and Muzio (2023).

Table 18.2   Causes of neonatal seizures.

Underlying cause	Condition	Information/examples
Hypoxia	Ischaemia	Blood oxygen depleted. Hypoxic-ischaemic encephalopathy
	Asphyxia	Oxygen depletion to lungs and brain
Thromboembolism	Arterial
Venous	Stroke
Thrombosis
Acute Metabolic disorder	Hypoglycaemia	May be linked to poor feeding
	Hypocalcaemia	May be linked to phototherapy
	Hypomagnesaemia
Hyponatraemia
Hypernatraemia	May be linked to incorrect feeding
Congenital Metabolic disorder	Enzyme deficiency	Urea cycle defect, diabetes, phenylketonuria
	Vitamin deficiency
Cofactor deficiency	Pyroxidine deficiency
Molybdenum cofactor deficiency
Haemorrhage	Intracranial
Intraventricular	
	Subarachnoid
Subdural
Intraparenchymal	
Acute infection	Bacterial meningitis	Group B *Streptococcus*, *Escherichia coli*
	Viral encephalitis	Herpes simplex
Congenital infection	Intrauterine	Toxoplasmosis, cytomegalovirus
Maternal drugs	Therapeutic	Maternal antipsychotic therapy
	Abuse	Neonatal opioid withdrawal syndrome
Epilepsy	Neonatal epilepsy syndromes	Benign seizures, congenital epilepsy
Brain malformations	Congenital structural abnormalities	Schizencephaly, holoprosencephaly, microcephaly, hydrocephaly
	Neonatal	Kernicterus

Source: Adapted from Krawiec and Muzio (2023).

Physical Examination of the Newborn at a Glance, Second Edition. Dr Lyn Dolby and Denise (Dee) Campbell.
© 2025 John Wiley & Sons Ltd. Published 2025 by John Wiley & Sons Ltd.

This chapter should be read in conjunction with those related to infection, neurological assessment, head, spine, cardiovascular and metabolic disorders. The examiner must be able to differentiate between physiological (e.g. benign neonatal sleep myoclonus) and pathological changes in body movements and tone. This will enable appropriate and timely referral. These symptoms are all relatively common but are often missed or misinterpreted.

Benign neonatal sleep myoclonus (Pachego and Singh, 2023)

This is a rare benign myoclonus that happens only during sleep in 4 : 10,000 births. Fast, repetitive jerks, involving some or all large limbs and the torso, occur multiple times. They are typically bilateral but less common in the face. They stop immediately a neonate wakes and typically resolve by 6 months. In most cases there is no links to opioid use, however they do occur more commonly in the neonates of mothers with addictions. In all cases, electroencephalogram (EEG) recordings will confirm these are not seizures.

Jitteriness

Jitteriness is a fast, intermittent tremor that mostly affects the limbs but less noticeably can affect the face and body. It results from excessive neuromuscular activity and the immaturity of the nervous system, and can be deliberately stimulated. In the majority of cases it is not associated with abnormality but is an over-active response to stimuli. Although more common with premature babies, it still occurs in around half of term newborns. Most often stopping within days, it can continue for months even when there is no pathological cause.

The Moro reflex may be mistaken for jitteriness.

Parents can also sometimes describe twitching during sleep as jitteriness, but these asymmetrical movements are normal during sleep. They are only a concern if prolonged or if cyanosis is observed.

To determine and confirm that an episode is jitteriness (and not any other pathological body movement) the examiner should try holding a limb (gently but firmly) and flexing the joint. If the tremor stops it is not any other form of seizure. It may also stop during sucking, so the sucking reflex can be stimulated and the tremor observed (see also Table 18.1). Jitteriness should appear:

- Symmetrical across the two sides of the body (never one sided).
- Rhythmic and gentle (no major jumping movement of the limbs).
- Without unusual eye, mouth or limb movements.
- Without change to breathing pattern or heart rate.

Confirmation that this is jitteriness (and not a seizure) does not automatically rule out complications. If this is an otherwise healthy newborn, feeding well, it was a brief episode and does not reoccur, then no further investigations will be required. However, if there are risk factors evident or the jitteriness is frequent and persistent, referral and further investigations are needed.

There are a number of conditions that may be associated with pathological jitteriness:

- Asphyxia.
- Hypernatraemia.
- Hypoglycaemia (the most common cause).
- Hypocalcaemia (risk increased during periods of phototherapy).
- Hypomagnesaemia.
- Intracranial haemorrhage.
- Sepsis.
- Withdrawal from maternal drugs such as antipsychotics or opioids (neonatal opioid withdrawal syndrome, previously known as fetal abstinence syndrome).

Seizures (convulsions or fits)

Electrical impulses within the brain can become over- or under-active when an imbalance in chemical changes occurs. A clinically apparent change in movement or tone occurs as a result and this is known as a seizure. Neonatal seizures can be provoked by acute brain injury or systemic insult, or may be unprovoked neonatal-onset epilepsy, where they are secondary to structural brain abnormalities, metabolic disorder or a genetic condition (Pisani et al., 2021; Ziobro and Shellhaas, 2020). The most common causes of provoked early-onset seizures are associated with hypoxic-ischaemic encephalopathy, asphyxia or stroke; later-onset seizures are more commonly associated with severe sepsis or intracranial haemorrhage (see Table 18.2 for a full list). Seizures remain commonly associated with neurological damage in infancy, linked to disability and mortality (Tanous et al., 2021).

The most common seizures during the first six weeks of life are subtle seizures where the clinical signs are often minor and frequently missed or confused with signs of hunger (see Box 18.1). Equally, these signs can be seen (even alongside generalised tonic movements) without EEG changes and therefore are not confirmed seizures. Continuous video EEG is the gold standard for diagnosis and monitoring of seizures (Carrasco and Stafstrom, 2024).

The other main seizures that are possible (see Box 18.2) may be accompanied by heart rate, respiration rate or blood pressure changes, as well as salivation and pupil changes. They can last for as little as 10 seconds to a number of minutes and come in quick succession or be minutes apart. After the subtle seizure, clonic and myoclonic seizures are the most likely. Tonic seizures are the rarest and are more common in pre-term infants (Sinha et al., 2018). The prognosis for the infant depends mostly on the underlying cause, with normal development least likely in the presence of structural abnormalities and bacterial meningitis and most likely in cases of hypocalcaemia, subarachnoid haemorrhage and an idiopathic cause (Sinha et al., 2018).

Hypotonia (floppiness)

This is when the newborn demonstrates a lack of muscle tone. That can be to varying degrees: localised (facial or Erb's palsy) or generalised (frog position), with or without evidence of muscle weakness. Tone decreases with degrees of prematurity but hypotonia is always abnormal in a term infant. The damage may be to the central or peripheral nervous system (e.g. asphyxia, trauma), muscles (e.g. congenital dystrophy) or a neuro-muscular junction (e.g. myasthenia gravis) (Sinha et al., 2018) (see Table 18.3). The condition may be temporary (e.g. metabolic or electrolyte disorder) or permanent (e.g. chromosomal condition or cerebral damage). Occasionally a condition can be associated with both seizures and hypotonia (e.g. hypoxic-ischaemic encephalopathy).

Congenital infection and neonatal sepsis

Table 19.1 Infections and their side effects.

Infection risk	Most common possible side effects for newborn
Candida albicans	Coated tongue and gums (white, creamy plaque), nappy rash
Conjunctivitis	Permanent scarring of the eye (secondary to *Staphylococcus aureus* and sexually transmitted infections).
Cytomegalovirus (CMV)	Microcephaly, hydrocephaly, cataract, chorioretinitis, hearing loss, organ disease, cerebral palsy, delayed development, brain calcification, rash (blueberry muffin spots)
Enterococcus faecalis	Skin and tissue infection, meningitis, conjunctivitis
Gonorrhoea	
Chlamydia	Conjunctivitis, profusely discharging eyes (ophthalmia)
Group B *Streptococcus* (GBS)	Septicaemia, pneumonia, meningitis, blindness, deafness, learning disability, lung weakness or even death
Hepatitis A, B and C	Chronic liver disease, cirrhosis, liver cancer
Herpes simplex virus (HSV)	Petechiae, infectious pustules, blisters and scarring, chorioretinitis, liver defects, anaemia, thrombocytopenia
Human immunodeficiency virus (HIV)	Intrauterine growth retardation (IUGR), microcephaly, facial defects (prominent forehead, triangular philtrum, enlarged lips)
Malaria	Fever, anaemia, splenomegaly, jaundice, loose stool, poor feeding
Meconium aspiration	Respiratory distress, cerebral irritability, pneumonitis, pneumothorax, hypoxia, acidosis, vascular necrosis, asphyxia or even death
Parvovirus B19	Slapped cheek facial rash, anaemia, eye defects, heart failure, hydrops fetalis
Rubella	IUGR, microcephaly, hydrocephaly, cataract, retinitis, glaucoma, deafness, heart defects, liver defects, hearing loss, rash (blueberry muffin spots), anaemia, bone weakness
Staphylococcus aureus	Yellow spots on skin, omphalitis, paronychia
Syphilis	IUGR, excoriating rash on palms of hands and soles of feet, changes in bone growth or development
Toxoplasmosis	IUGR, microcephaly, hydrocephaly, cataract, retinitis, deafness, heart defects, liver defects, hearing loss, rash, anaemia, brain calcification
Treponema pallidum	Hydrocephalus, deafness, bone defects, developmental defects
Tuberculosis (TB)	Fever, respiratory problems, pneumonia
Varicella zoster virus (VZV; chickenpox)	Eye damage, microcephaly, defects in the brain or spine (causing hypoplasia or partial paralysis), skin excoriation and scarring, urogenital defects

The newborn is at risk from various sources of infection. These may have been transplacental, ascending uterine, intrapartum, through feeds or via direct contact after birth. While many maternal infections do not affect the fetus, the ones that do increase both morbidity and mortality through miscarriage, premature labour, growth retardation or developmental abnormalities. All infections should be treated as significant due to the potential side effects and the possibility of a rapid decline in newborn health. They must be managed without delay, including early (and possibly urgent) referral for full investigation and septic screen.

Risk factors

There are a number of maternal risk factors that will increase the risk of congenitally acquired infections. Some of these are routinely screened for in pregnancy, while others may be screened for after identification of increased risk. The maternal history should be reviewed for evidence of any of the following:
- Viral infection, e.g. human immunodeficiency virus (HIV), rubella, CMV, parvovirus, herpes simplex virus (HSV), varicella zoster virus (VZV).
- Sexually transmitted disease, e.g. syphilis, chlamydia, gonorrhoea.
- Bacterial infection, e.g. group B *Streptococcus* (GBS).
- Fungal infection, e.g. *Candida albicans*.
- Maternal rash, malaise or 'flu-like' symptoms.
- Antibodies detected during serology screening.
- Maternal pyrexia.
- Pre-term and/or prolonged rupture of membranes.
- Meconium liquor.
- Chorioamnionitis.
- Substance misuse.
- Previous infant with GBS.
- Toxoplasmosis (parasite) screening.

Following birth, the sepsis risk is increased in the presence of the following:
- Maternal infection, e.g. mastitis.
- Inappropriate hygiene standards.
- Maternal learning disability (affecting hygiene standards).
- Exposure to sibling, partner or visitor infection.
- Prematurity.
- Hospital delivery – environment, staff and equipment.
- Invasive procedures (and prolonged labours).

Signs and symptoms

Information should be gleaned from the patterns of sleeping, feeding and if there has been any vomiting. This should reveal the following:
- Any unusual drowsiness or an unresponsive baby.
- Infrequent or poor feeding.
- Poor weight gain (at the six-week examination).
- Vomiting.

In addition, the practitioner should look for signs of the following:
- Tachypnoea, bradypnoea, chest recession, grunting or apnoea (often the first or an early sign of sepsis).
- Abnormalities linked to congenital infections.
- Haematuria (ensure this is not pseudo-menstruation or urates).
- Inflammation, redness or an area of localised heat.
- Pallor or a mottled appearance.
- Delayed perfusion (poor capillary refill time).
- Localised serous fluid leak, septic spots or any purulent exudate.
- Diarrhoea or dehydration.
- Systemic temperature that is low, raised (above 38 °C) or unstable.
- High-pitched cry.
- Hypo- or hypertonia, jitteriness or seizures.
- Hypo- or hyperglycaemia.
- An area of swelling and/or tenderness.
- Bradycardia or tachycardia.
- Jaundice or enlarged liver.
- Acidosis or shock.

Management

Any high-risk or symptomatic newborn should have been managed accordingly. The practitioner must review the results of any of the following:
- Regular observations of respiration efforts, temperature, heart rate, colour, behaviour, responsiveness and oxygen saturation. The NEWTT2 risk identification and observational chart (British Association of Perinatal Medicine, 2024) complements clinical skills.
- Septic screen (swabs, urine or stool samples, blood samples or cerebrospinal fluid from lumbar puncture).
- Monitoring of fluid balance including feeding and excretion.

Where significant sepsis has been confirmed, antibiotic treatment and admission to a NICU will have been likely for respiratory and cardiovascular support, thermoregulation, fluid/feed supplementation, medications and 24-hour monitoring.

Specific infections and their side effects

Many of the possible neonatal infections are listed in Table 19.1 along with their side effects. The two most commonly occurring are expanded on next.

Group B Streptococcus

GBS is the most common cause of newborn sepsis and has the potential to be fatal. Bacteria colonises the maternal vaginal tract, introducing the risk of ascending infection (when there is prolonged rupture of the membranes) and contact during delivery. It can also be passed on in breastmilk or by a carer. Preventative management includes intrapartum antibiotics (at least two hours before delivery) followed by regular observation of temperature and respirations after birth. Unmanaged, the risks to the newborn are as follows:
- Respiratory distress and/or pneumonia.
- Septicaemia.
- Meningitis.

These can progress to blindness, deafness, learning disability, lung weakness or even death.

Conjunctivitis

Redness of the conjunctiva, purulent discharge and oedema of one or both eyes are strong indicators of infection. The most common causes relate to a blocked lachrymal duct, *Staphylococcus aureus* or contact with a sexually transmitted infection during birth. Of greatest concern is ophthalmia identified at the first examination caused by *Neisseria gonorrhoeae* (occurring within 24 hours of birth), which can cause permanent scarring if management is delayed. Chlamydial and syphilitic infections will typically present later.

20 Anaemia and polycythaemia

Figure 20.1 Fetal red cells reduced – anaemia.
Source: Reproduced with permission from Lissauer et al. (2020)/John Wiley & Sons.

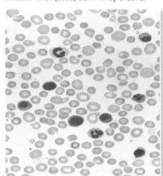

Figure 20.2 Maternal cells mixed with fetal haemoglobin.
Source: Reproduced with permission from Lissauer et al. (2020)/John Wiley & Sons.

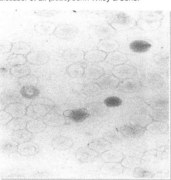

Fetomaternal hemorrhage (Figure 20.1). Anaemia (number of red cells are reduced), nucleated red cells (erythroblasts) and reticulocytes on a blood smear (film) from a term neonate with severe anaemia at birth (4.5 g/dL) caused by fetomaternal haemorrhage.

(Figure 20.2) Kleihauer test on maternal blood from the same baby showing several intensely pink-stained cells containing HbF, which is resistant to acid lysis

Figure 20.3 Causes and investigations of anaemia – with and without jaundice complication.
Source: Reproduced with permission from Lissauer et al. (2020)/John Wiley & Sons.

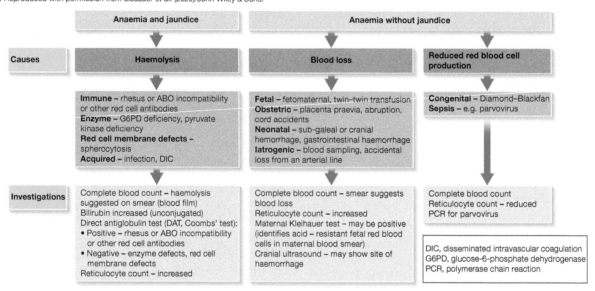

	Anaemia and jaundice	Anaemia without jaundice	
Causes	Haemolysis	Blood loss	Reduced red blood cell production
	Immune – rhesus or ABO incompatibility or other red cell antibodies **Enzyme** – G6PD deficiency, pyruvate kinase deficiency **Red cell membrane defects** – spherocytosis **Acquired** – infection, DIC	**Fetal** – fetomaternal, twin–twin transfusion **Obstetric** – placenta praevia, abruption, cord accidents **Neonatal** – sub-galeal or cranial hemorrhage, gastrointestinal haemorrhage **Iatrogenic** – blood sampling, accidental loss from an arterial line	**Congenital** – Diamond–Blackfan **Sepsis** – e.g. parvovirus
Investigations	Complete blood count – haemolysis suggested on smear (blood film) Bilirubin increased (unconjugated) Direct antiglobulin test (DAT, Coombs' test): • Positive – rhesus or ABO incompatibility or other red cell antibodies • Negative – enzyme defects, red cell membrane defects Reticulocyte count – increased	Complete blood count – smear suggests blood loss Reticulocyte count – increased Maternal Kleihauer test – may be positive (identifies acid – resistant fetal red blood cells in maternal blood smear) Cranial ultrasound – may show site of haemorrhage	Complete blood count Reticulocyte count – reduced PCR for parvovirus

DIC, disseminated intravascular coagulation
G6PD, glucose-6-phosphate dehydrogenase
PCR, polymerase chain reaction

Figure 20.4 Oxygen affinity of neonatal haemoglobin versus adult haemoglobin.
Source: Reproduced with permission from Lissauer et al. (2020)/John Wiley & Sons.

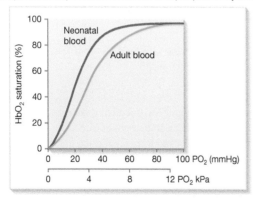

Figure 20.5 Plethoric newborn (nasogastric tube associated with poor feeding).
Source: Reproduced with permission from Lissauer et al. (2020)/John Wiley & Sons.

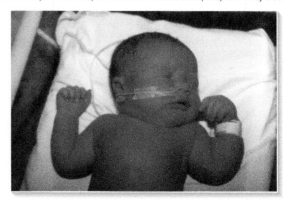

Delayed cord clamping

This chapter aims to help the examiner understand anaemia and polycythaemia, in order to enable recognition of risk factors, signs and symptoms. The most debated contributing factor is **delayed cord clamping**. The blood volume of a newborn ranges from 75 to 100 mL/kg. Delayed cord clamping can increase this by as much as 25–30%, with the benefit of reducing the likelihood of both physiological and iron-deficiency anaemia. However, the increased circulating blood volume and potential concentration of RBCs can also increase the risk of polycythaemia and jaundice. The Resuscitation Council UK (2021) guidelines recommend delaying cord clamping for at least one minute for all healthy newborn infants and for up to three minutes for premature births. This assumes that resuscitation is not required and maternal consent has been given.

Anaemia

Neonatal anaemia is defined by the reduced level of circulating haemoglobin (Figure 20.1). Haemoglobin consists of red pigmented haem (containing ferrous iron) and the protein globin. It performs the essential roles of transporting oxygen around the various cells of the body. Lower levels of circulating oxygen in utero necessitate a high fetal haemoglobin level and higher oxygen affinity (Figure 20.4). This remains high for the neonate for 6–8 weeks after birth, with a normal range from 140 to 220 g/L. Below 100 g/L is considered to be anaemia with below 80 g/L considered severe. Anaemia may occur in either of the following situations:

- **Haemorrhage**: may occur in utero, at or after birth.
- **Reduction in red cells**: under-production or excessive destruction (Figure 20.3).

Predisposing factors

Ironically, the most common cause for anaemia is induced through repeated blood sampling from premature infants. Other factors are associated with haemorrhage and include the following:

- **Placental trauma**: abruption, praevia, chorionic villi sampling (CVS), trauma during surgery, vasa praevia, snapped cord.
- **Fetomaternal transfusion**: CVS, amniocentesis, abdominal trauma (raised Kleihauer present, see Figure 20.2).
- **Twin–twin transfusion**: one twin anaemic, the other polycythaemic.
- **Birth trauma**: fracture, bruising, cephalhaematoma, sub-galeal haematoma, abdominal or chest compression.
- **Abnormality**: gastrointestinal bleeding.

Physiological reduction of the haemoglobin occurs naturally after birth to reduce the high level inherited from fetal life. Pathological destruction, under-production and abnormalities in formation are also possible, associated with the following risk factors:

- **Uterine hypoxia**: meconium in utero, sinusoidal electronic cardiotocography (ECTG), fetal blood gases, fetal compromise.
- **Placental insufficiency**: growth-deficient fetus or newborn.
- **Maternal disease**: diabetes, disseminated intravascular coagulation, autoimmune disease.
- **Congenital infection**.
- **Genetic disease**: Diamond-Blackfan, G6PD, thalassaemia.
- **Blood cell disorders**: pyknocytosis, spherocytosis.
- **Haemolysis**: Rhesus or ABO incompatibility (antibodies, positive Coombs' test), sibling anaemia.
- **Dietary deficiency**: vitamin E or iron.
- **Hormone imbalance**: reduction in, or lack of, erythropoietin.

Most common early signs and symptoms, with management

- Pale.
- Lethargic.
- Poor feeding or failure to thrive.
- Tachycardia.
- Tachypnoea (deteriorating to intermittent apnoea).
- Enlarged liver.
- Jaundice.

Oral folic acid and iron therapy management should be considered (particularly pre-term), but are unlikely to be required when formula feeding (contains supplements). Blood transfusion thresholds vary but aim to balance hazards against clinical significance.

Polycythaemia

This is a condition of excessive RBCs or high packed cell volume (haematocrit). The percentage of packed cells to whole blood at birth ranges from 55 to 68%, peaking at 6–12 hours old due to haemoconcentration, and dropping to 32–45% by 6 weeks old. Polycythaemia is relatively common at levels above 65%. Polycythaemia does not automatically mean that blood becomes viscous, but this will complicate almost half of cases when microthrombi may develop and block smaller blood vessels. Polycythaemia is associated with the following conditions:

- Increased red cell production (erythropoietin).
- Increased blood volume.

Predisposing factors

- **Hypoxic episodes stimulate compensatory red cell increase for oxygen carrying capacity**: placental abruption, maternal smoker, placental insufficiency, poor fetal growth, post-date pregnancy.
- **Excessive placental transfusion**: delayed cord clamping, twin–twin transfusion, gravity (infant below placental height).
- **Maternal disease**: diabetic mother, gestational diabetes, pre-eclampsia, heart disease, renal disease.
- **Newborn disease**: endocrine abnormalities linked to fetal hypoxia (thyrotoxicosis, Beckwith-Wiedemann syndrome, hyperglycaemia).
- **Newborn genetic disorders**: trisomies 13, 18 or 21, diabetes.

Most common early signs and symptoms, with management

Many polycythaemic newborns are asymptomatic but signs increase with the degree of problem:

- Normal colour at rest, plethoric when distressed (Figure 20.5).
- Sleepiness and poor feeding.
- Irritability on handling.
- Oliguria and/or haematuria.
- Jitteriness and tremors, progressing to seizures.
- Thrombosis and cerebrovascular accidents.
- Tachypnoea (respiratory disease and intermittent apnoea).
- Cyanosis (rare as a neonate), progressing to heart failure.
- Priapism (male infants).
- Hypo- or hyper-glycaemia.
- Jaundice and hyper-bilirubinaemia.
- Necrotising enterocolitis.
- Thrombocytopenia.

Partial exchange transfusion (blood replaced by 0.9% saline) is avoided but may be needed if symptoms are clinically significant, or haematocrit has reached 70%.

21 Genetics and inheritance

Figure 21.1 Chromosomes and genes.

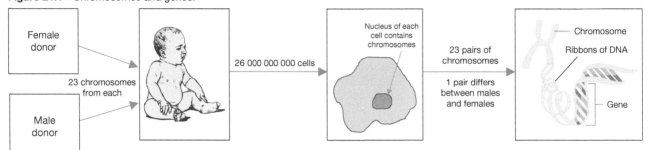

Figure 21.2 Autosomal dominant inheritance (e.g. diabetes mellitus type 1).
Source: (Top) Lakhani et al. (2024)/John Wiley & Sons. (Bottom) Cancer Research UK/ https://upload.wikimedia.org/wikipedia/commons/4/43/Diagram_of_a_gene_on_a_ chromosome_CRUK_020.svg, last accessed 11 May 2024/Wikipedia/CC BY 4.0.

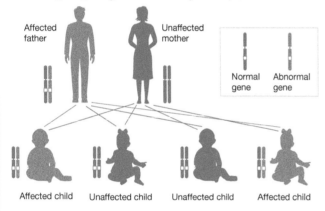

Figure 21.3 Autosomal recessive inheritance (e.g. diabetes mellitus type 1).
Source: (Top) Lakhani et al. (2024)/John Wiley & Sons. (Bottom) Cancer Research UK/ https://upload.wikimedia.org/wikipedia/commons/4/43/Diagram_of_a_gene_on_a_ chromosome_CRUK_020.svg, last accessed 11 May 2024 / Wikipedia/CC BY 4.0.

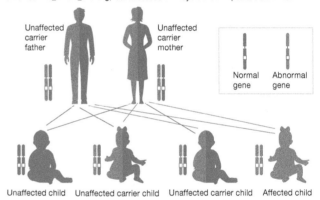

Figure 21.4 X-Linked dominant inheritance (e.g. vitamin D-resistant rickets).
Source: Lakhani et al. (2024)/John Wiley & Sons.

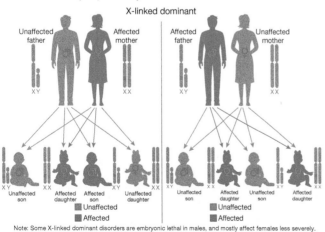

Note: Some X-linked dominant disorders are embryonic lethal in males, and mostly affect females less severely.

Figure 21.5 X-Linked recessive inheritance (e.g. haemophilia).
Source: Lakhani et al. (2024)/John Wiley & Sons.

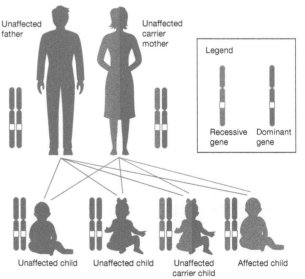

This chapter aims to increase understanding around terminology, chromosomes, genetics and inheritance. The practitioner must appreciate that not all families involve a mother, father and dual parenting. Fertility support enables single-sex parenting and this requires sensitivity around referring to sperm donors as fathers, surrogates as parents, or the child of a rape victim as having a father. Ensure you know any terminology preferences before discussing familial or genetic histories.

Antenatal risk factors, screening and diagnostics

Risk factors at booking include age, family history, alcoholism, diabetes, thyroidism, drug misuse and carrier status. Antenatal screening for fetal genetic abnormalities includes nuchal translucency, hormone levels (triple and quadruple blood tests) and scanning (soft markers). Diagnostic analysis of fetal cells may occur through amniocentesis (amniotic liquor), cordocentesis (fetal blood), CVS or the less invasive analysis of fetal cell-free DNA (cfDNA) from a maternal blood sample.

The two main methods of testing chromosomes are karyotyping and fluorescent in-situ hybridisation (FISH). Karyotyping is testing of the entire set of chromosomes. It is the 'gold standard' but takes up to two weeks and is only possible for less than 10% of samples. FISH, by comparison, is a relatively rapid technique for locating specific DNA sequences on a chromosome and diagnosing genetic disease, but it has high false-positive and false-negative rates (Queremel Milani and Tadi, 2024).

Cytogenetics and genetics

Cytogenetics is the study of chromosomes from samples of tissue, blood or blood marrow. Genetics is the study of individual genes along these chromosomes. Both analyse the part they play in disease and inheritance. Every human trait and disease has a genetic basis, with environmental factors such as lifestyle and diet also having an impact.

Cells, chromosomes, genes and DNA

The body of a newborn is made up of 9,000,000,000 cells and each cell has a different specialised function. The nuclei of most of these cells contain 23 pairs of chromosomes (half from the male donor and half from the female donor). These typically consist of 22 autosomes (any chromosome that is not a sex chromosome) and one pair of sex chromosomes (XX or XY), but ova and sperm are haploid (containing just one copy of each chromosome). Chromosomes are made up of ribbons of deoxyribonucleic acid (DNA) and along this 2 m ribbon are the 20–25,000 genes (Figure 21.1). Cells use these genes selectively. The elaborate DNA within the genes contains hereditary information as codes, for the production of specific proteins and to enable cells to perform different functions.

Genetic testing and genetic variants

Genetic disorders occur when the DNA sequence changes and individual genes do not function normally. Genetic testing analyses changes in a selected group of genes for genetic variants, plus it assesses if they affect both chromosomes of the pair:

- **Homozygous**: same variant detected on both copies of the gene.
- **Heterozygous**: variant only present on one copy of the gene.
- **Hemizygous**: only one copy of the gene and it contains the variant.
  Genetic variants are not always associated with a disorder. They can be assigned to one of five classifications (Lakhani et al., 2024):
- **Pathogenic (Class 5)**: affects gene function causing a genetic disorder.
- **Likely pathogenic (Class 4)**: probably affects gene function; likely to cause a genetic disorder.

- **Variant of uncertain significance (Class 3)**: insufficient information to know if the variant causes a disorder.
- **Unlikely pathogenic/likely benign (Class 2)**: probably a normal genetic variant; unlikely to cause a disorder.
- **Not pathogenic/benign (Class 1)**: known to be a normal variant in the population that does not cause disorders.

Genetic disorders and inheritance

Genetic factors play a part in nearly all health conditions. When a genetic change is exclusively responsible this is known as a genetic disorder or inherited disease. There are believed to be over 6000 known genetic disorders. Genetic disease divides into three major groups (Queremel Milani and Tadi, 2024):

- **Single-gene (mutations)**: a single gene is affected; can be either a natural variation in DNA (polymorphism) or result in an altered protein. The mutation can be a missing, duplicated, inserted or deleted gene affecting ability to function. Cell performance can be reduced or disabled or can malfunction and the effect is contingent on how important that gene is for survival. Single-gene mutations affect 1 : 50 people.

The genes affected can be found on the autosomal chromosomes (numbers 1–22) or on the sex chromosomes (mostly X linked). Inheritance depends on the location of the gene and whether one or two copies are needed for normal functioning. There are five inheritance patterns for single gene disorders (Figures 21.2, 21.3, 21.4 and 21.5):

- **Autosomal dominant** (Figure 21.2): all individuals carrying the mutated gene are affected; it is not possible to be an unaffected carrier. Examples are achondroplasia, osteogenesis imperfecta.
- **Autosomal recessive** (Figure 21.3): affected individuals must have two copies of the gene; carriers will have one copy of the gene. Examples are cystic fibrosis, PKU, thalassaemia, sickle cell anaemia.
- **X-linked dominant** (Figure 21.4): females more frequently affected; no male-to-male transmission. Examples are vitamin D-resistant rickets, incontinentia pigmenti.
- **X-linked recessive** (Figure 21.5): males more frequently affected; can only pass to a daughter if both donors are carriers. Examples are haemophilia, Duchenne muscular dystrophy, G6PDD.
- **Mitochondrial**: only females can pass the condition on, but both males and females are affected. Example is Leigh syndrome.
- **Chromosomal**: usually an error in cell division (mitosis or miosis) affecting more than one gene and causing either a change in numbers of chromosomes (numerical), e.g. aneuploidy (most common are trisomies 13, 18 and 21), or a change in structure (structural), e.g. deletions, translocations, insertions, inversions and duplications of a segment.
- **Multifactorial**: a combination of genetic, behavioural (e.g. diet, smoking, drugs) and environmental factors (e.g. pollution, metals), including diabetes, cancer and heart disease.

Indicators of genetic disorder

- Antenatal diagnostic test result, e.g. trisomies 13, 18 or 21.
- Post-natal screening or diagnostic test result, e.g. cystic fibrosis.
- Family history of genetic disorders, e.g. thalassaemia.
- Physical birth defects, e.g. cataracts, cleft lip or palate, congenital heart disease, diaphragmatic hernia, spina bifida, missing digits/limbs, dysmorphic features, single palmar crease, simian crease, epicanthic folds, different-coloured eyes, head circumference, large or small tongue, ear abnormalities, webbed digits, birthmark, absence of testes.
- Poor feeding, vomiting and failure to thrive, e.g. PKU.
- Hypotonia and poor activity, e.g. muscular dystrophy, trisomy 21.
- Seizures, e.g. benign familial neonatal epilepsy.

22 Syndromes and signs

Achondroplasia (dwarfism)

Megalocephaly
Prominent forehead
Protruding jaw
Flat area between eyes
Short limbs
Kyphosis
Lordosis
Associated with hydrocephalus,
upper airway obstruction

Beckwith-Weidemann

Macrosomia
Asymmetrical growth
Macroglossia
Ear creases or pits
Associated with omphalocele,
hernias, hypoglycaemia,
enlarged abdominal organs,
cancerous and non-cancerous
tumours (Wilms tumour)

CHARGE

C= Coloboma (hole/defect of eye)
H= Heart defects
A= Atresia Choanae
R= Restricted growth/develoment
G= Genitourinary abnormalities
E= Ear abnormalities

Crouzan

Early fusion of sutures/
fontanelles/facial bones
Brachycephaly
Wide-set, bulging eyes
Strabismus
Beak-like nose
Flattened cheeks
Protruding chin
Low-set ears
Under-developed upper jaw
Concave face
Short humerus and femur
Associated with narrow ear
canal, heart defects, cleft
lip/palate

Cornelia de Lange

Low birth weight/slow growth
Microcephaly
Excessive body hair
Thin, arched, joined eyebrows
Low-set ears
Long eyelashes
Narrow downturned lips
Upturned nose
(Mild forms have no signs)
Associated with cleft palate,
gastrointestinal problems,
seizures, heart defects, eye
problems

Cri du chat

High-pitched, cat-like cry
Hypotonia
Low birth weight/slow growth
Microcephaly
Downward slant to wide-set eyes
Epicanthic folds
Low-set ears
Abnormally shaped/folding ears
Micrognathia
Single palmar crease
Associated with inguinal hernia,
diastasis recti

Downs (trisomy 21)

Hypotonia
Flat occiput
Third fontanelle
Upward-slanting eyes
Epicanthic folds
Low-set ears
Simple pinna
Short neck
Single palmar crease (Simian
line)
Short little finger
Wide space between first and
second toes
Associated with omphalocele,
duodenal atresia, heart
disease, Hirschsprung disease

Edwards (trisomy 18)

Low birth weight
High mortality rate
Microcephaly
Micrognathia
Small mouth
Low-set ears
Long overlapping fingers
Under-developed thumbs
Clenched fists
Smooth, 'rocker bottom' feet
Kyphosis
Associated with cleft lip and
palate, cardiac and kidney
disease, hernias, exomphalos,
talipes, bone abnormalities,
urinary infections

Fetal alcohol (FA)

Low birth weight
Reduced head circumference
Small eye openings
Epicanthal folds
Short palpebral fissure
Flat mid-face
Minor ear abnormalities
Short nose
Thin upper lip
Indistinct philtrum
Micrognathia

Klippel-Feil

Fusion of 2+ cervical vertebrae
Limited neck movement
Shorter neck
Low hairline
Elevated scapulae (Sprengel
deformity)
Scoliosis
Asymmetrical limb lengths
Associated with heart, lung,
kidney, genito-urinary
deformities; cleft palate;
spina bifida

Goldenhar (oculo-auricular-vertebral, OAV) or hemifacial macrosomia

Incomplete development of eyes, ears, nose, soft palate, lip and
mandible – small, missing or misshapen parts, skin tags, strabismus
Hemifacial macrosomia
Fused or missing vertebrae
Scoliosis
Associated with deafness, blindness, heart defects, breathing and
feeding difficulties, limbal dermoids (eye tumours)

Marfan's

Connective tissue disorder
Longer limbs and fingers
Scoliosis
High palate
Long, narrow face
Associated with heart, bones, joints, lung, eyes, skin and blood vessel disorders

Neonatal abstinence

Amount and type of alcohol/drug withdrawal
Low birth weight, poor weight gain
Mottled colouring
Hypertonic
Hyperactive reflexes
High-pitched, frequent crying
Loose stool
Vomiting
Fever
Irritability, jitteriness, seizures
Excessive suck but poor feeder
Sweating
Associated with maternal alcohol or drug dependence

Pierre-Robin

Retrognathia (abnormal jaw or maxilla)
Micrognathia (small lower jaw)
Glossoptosis (tongue falls back)
Natal teeth
Associated with difficulty breathing; cleft, holed or high-arched palate; large tongue; a second syndrome, e.g. FAS

Turners

Low birth weight
Females only
Swollen hands
Thick neck tissue
Associated with infertility, heart and kidney abnormalities

Mermaid (sirenomelia)

Legs fused together
Associated with kidney, bladder, bowel and genitalia abnormalities; typically mortality within 48 hours

Noonan

Large head compared to face
Tall forehead
Epicanthal folds
Downward-slanting palpebral fissure
Short, broad nose
Deep philtrum
Full lips
Micrognathia
Low-set, thickened ears
Posteriorly rotated, oval ears
Oedema of hands and feet
Webbed neck – excess nuchal skin
Sunken sternum
Associated with heart defects

Poland

Concave chest (absent or reduced muscle)
Abnormal or short ribs
Nipple abnormalities
Short radius and ulna on affected side
Abnormal hand on same side – webbed or fused fingers
Associated with Sprengel deformity, facial paralysis, leukaemia, non-Hodgkin lymphoma

Treacher Collins

Absent malar bones
Under-developed jaw
Downward-slanting eyes
Micrognathia
Abnormal ears
Associated with cleft palate, respiratory problems, deafness, droopy appearance

Nail-patella

Affects nails, bones, kidneys, eyes
Small, poorly developed nails
Patellar aplasia – absent, small or luxated
Elbows misshaped
Scoliosis
Cervical ribs present
Abnormal scapulae

Patau (trisomy 13)

Low birth weight
Hypotelorism or cyclops
Cleft lip and palate
Small eyes
Malformed nose
Neural tube defects
Microcephaly
Ear malformations
Polydactyly
Rocker-bottom feet
Associated with heart, kidney and gastrointestinal defects; deafness; holoprosencephaly, feeding problems

Prader-Willi

Hypotonia
Weak reflexes
Poor suck reflex/poor feeder
Almond-shaped eyes
Small hands and feet
Weak cry
Thin upper lip
Downturned mouth
Hypogonadism
Scoliosis
Associated with one or more undescended testes

Zellweger

Hypotonia
Wide-set eyes
Under-developed eyebrow ridges
Poor suck and swallow
Enlarged liver
Seizures
Associated with jaundice, gastrointestinal bleeding

23 Intrapartum trauma and injury

Figure 23.1 Equipment injuries.

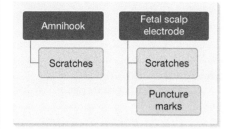

Table 23.1 Incidence of common types of birth injury.

Type of birth injury and approximate incidence		NOTE: The incident levels given are approximations. This is due to a number of factors that may be present at the time of delivery, for example the expertise of the practitioner responsible at the time of the delivery, type of instrumental equipment used, maternal factors (obesity etc.), neonatal factors (prematurity, large baby etc.). Also, the incident rate will vary across countries in association with birth practices/policy and reporting systems. Therefore, it is prudent to investigate your local and national statistics.
Cephalhaematoma	2 : 100	
Facial nerve palsy	2 : 1000	
Brachial plexus injury	0.5 : 1000	
Subaponeurotic haemorrhage	1 : 1250	
Major subdural haemorrhage	1.1 : 50,000	
Skull fractures	Rare	
Spinal cord injuries	Very rare	

Figure 23.2 Areas of extracranial and intercranial haemorrhage.
Source: Brosansky et al. (2021)/Reproduced with permission of Elsevier.

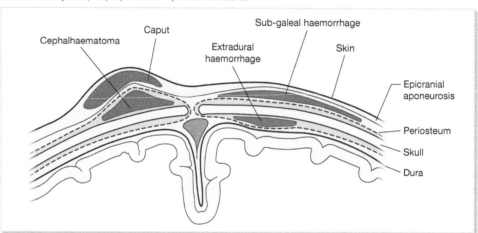

Table 23.2 Brachial plexus injury.

Cause	Excessive lateral flexion, rotation or traction of the neonatal neck at delivery Unexplained – possible prenatal cause
Erb's palsy	Where the arm lies adducted in the classic waiter's tip position but movement of the fingers is retained
Klumpke's palsy	More likely to occur in pre-term infants during a difficult delivery of the head during a breech delivery It involves the small muscles of the hand with accompanying wrist drop and flaccid paralysis of the hand, resulting in an absent grasp reflex
Total paralysis of the arm	Trauma has occurred to all trunks of the brachial plexus, resulting in flaccidity of the arm Cutis marmorata may be visible as a result of vasomotor disturbance In the event of bilateral impact, spinal injury should be suspected

Physical Examination of the Newborn at a Glance, Second Edition. Dr Lyn Dolby and Denise (Dee) Campbell.
© 2025 John Wiley & Sons Ltd. Published 2025 by John Wiley & Sons Ltd.

At or soon after birth, particular minor abnormalities or birth injuries may be observed. Some may have occurred during the passage of the fetus through the bony pelvis. Others may be the result of the use of equipment (Figure 23.1) or of instrumental delivery due to poor application or inappropriate force being applied when using forceps/ventouse, or as the consequence of urgent actions performed during delivery (e.g. shoulder dystocia). The incidence of common birth injuries is given in Table 23.1.

Soft tissue injury

• **Traumatic petechiae** can be visualised from head to upper chest, usually as the result of a difficult delivery. They may be mistaken for cyanosis but O$_2$ saturation will be normal. They commonly occur with breech delivery or when the umbilical cord is wound tightly round the neonatal neck, resulting in a sudden increase in intrathoracic pressure as the chest compresses at delivery. Petechiae in this instance are transitory, usually fading within 2–3 days. They must not be confused with generalised petechiae across the body, which are associated with low platelets or coagulopathy.

• **Bruising** may result from a precipitate or traumatic birth as the result of abnormal presentation (e.g. face, brow or breech) or in the presence of thrombocytopenia. Parents should be informed that depending on the degree of bruising, jaundice is more likely because of the increased bilirubin breakdown.

• **Subcutaneous fat necrosis** is an obvious induration of the skin caused by pressure being applied to the skin, either in utero or externally (e.g. bony pelvis, forceps blades).

Extracranial and intercranial trauma

Figure 23.2 gives a diagrammatic representation of where haemorrhage for the following conditions occurs:

• **Cephalhaematoma** is the result of repeated contact between the fetal skull and the maternal pelvis, although pressure caused during vacuum delivery can also be a factor. Shearing of the veins between the periosteum and cranial bones (usually the parietal region but occasionally occipital) causes bleeding, the extent of which is limited by the suture lines. Gentle palpation of the area will assist in detecting any underlying skull fracture. The subperiosteal bleeding is slow and may not be visible until some hours or days later, when it eventually reaches its fullest extent. Swelling may persist for several weeks. Parents should be informed of the increased risk of jaundice.

• **Subaponeurotic (or subgaleal) haemorrhage** is most often but not exclusively seen in highly pigmented infants. This rare type of haemorrhage is the result of bleeding occurring beneath the aponeurotic sheet that joins the parts of the occipitofrontalis muscle. Causative factors include trauma during delivery (e.g. vacuum extraction) or it may be the result of a coagulation disorder (Yim et al., 2023). Rapid swelling produces the 'hot water bottle' sign, where the scalp feels fluctuant when palpated. Blood loss can be acute and under-estimated, with haemoglobin levels falling significantly, resulting in neonatal shock. Rapid diagnosis and appropriate management with fluid replacement in the first instance are paramount (Fanning, 2024).

• **Intercranial haemorrhage** may occur as a direct consequence of trauma, but is more often the result of hypoxic–ischaemic injury. Encephalopathy or seizures may be present and immediate neonatal consultant management is required on recognition.

Bone and joint injuries

• **Skull fracture** may be associated with forceps delivery or, more rarely, head compression with the maternal sacral promontory. Linear fractures usually require no treatment, but depressed or large fractures may indicate underlying trauma and neurosurgical consultation should be sought. Depressed skull fractures can take some months to resolve post birth.

• **Fracture of the clavicle**, the most frequent bone to be fractured, usually associated with shoulder dystocia or a difficult breech delivery. As with adults, management is minimal, with the offer of pain relief if the baby appears uncomfortable.

• **Fractured humerus or femur** occurs rarely, usually as a result of trauma during delivery. Immobilisation is the care management of choice. Radial nerve injury can sometimes occur with the former and integrity of the nerve supply should be assessed.

• **Multiple fractures** are rare and therefore the possibility of osteogenesis imperfecta should be explored.

• **Unusual fractures**, occurring after birth or after the baby has been discharged home, should always be investigated. Parents need to be cared for sensitively as the inference is often of a non-accidental injury. Provision of an accurate account from both the parents and the healthcare professionals at the time is paramount. If no immediate cause is clearly apparent, social services and the police are often involved. Reviewing and gaining an understanding of the safeguarding policies within one's own NHS Trust is invaluable.

Peripheral nerve trauma

Generally, the most likely nerve trauma to be found is the result of a *brachial plexus injury*, which has a strong association with shoulder dystocia. However, nerve trauma can also occur during delivery of the after-coming head in a breech presentation. The three types of paralysis are highlighted in Table 23.2:

• **Facial nerve palsy**, when oblique application of forceps blades or prolonged pressure within the bony pelvis may result in an inability to close the eye and a lack of expression on the affected side when the baby cries. In most cases recovery occurs by 6 weeks of age.

• **Radial nerve trauma** is rarely seen in practice, but may result from a fracture of the humerus if there is difficulty in delivery of the arm during a breech delivery. Previously, giving an intramuscular injection into the deltoid region was associated with radial nerve damage, which is why this area is now avoided for injection.

• **Other rarer forms of nerve trauma** include sciatic and phrenic nerve injury, recurrent laryngeal nerve and spinal cord injury.

Organ injuries: liver, spleen, kidneys and testes

A traumatic breech delivery (or, rarely, an atraumatic vertex delivery) can cause subcapsular haematoma of the liver. In the event of hepatosplenomegaly (rhesus haemolytic disease, mother with diabetes), rupture of the liver or spleen may have already occurred. Rupture of the kidneys can also occur in pre-term infants who present breech at delivery.

Adrenal haemorrhage may occur with breech deliveries, but an overwhelming bacterial infection of disseminated intravascular coagulopathy is most likely to be the cause. Bruising of the testes may be seen in breech deliveries and is usually treated with analgesia.

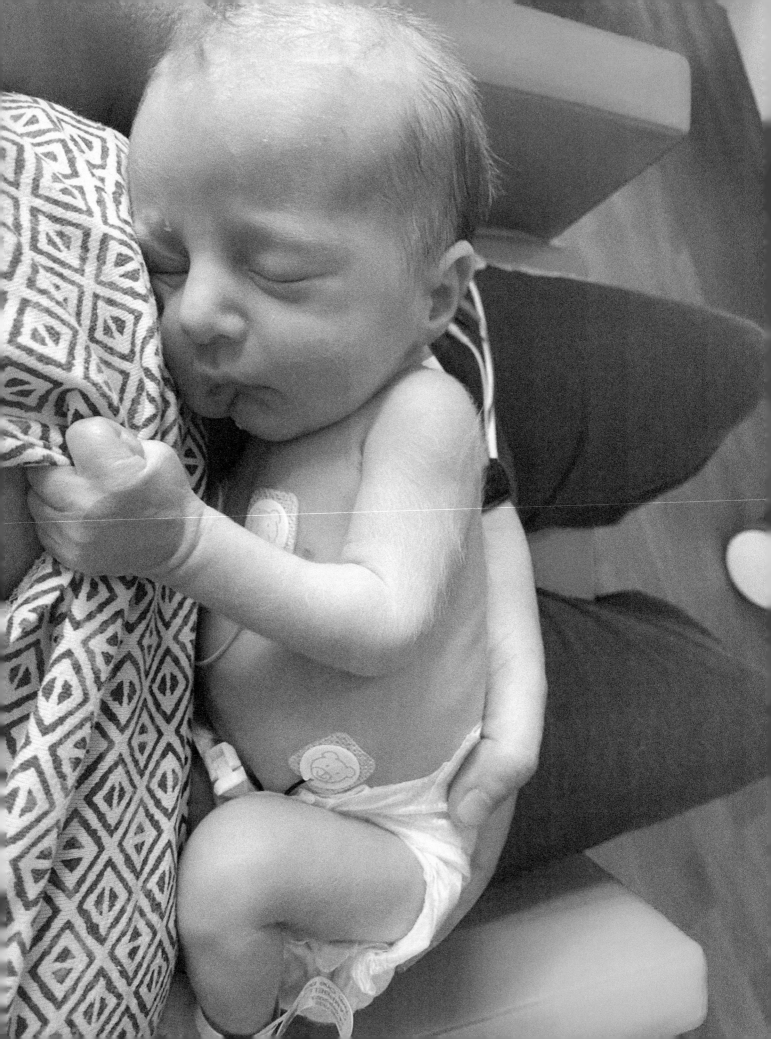

Allied assessments

Part 3

Chapters

24 Initial examination at birth: overview

Table 24.1 Key areas of assessment in the initial newborn examination.

Aspect	Investigate prior information, observe and assess the following elements	
Predisposing factors	Investigate *Recorded history*: family, antenatal, intrapartum and maternal/neonatal progress or concerns since birth *Ask parent(s)*: for information on any concerns or family history relevant to their baby that they wish to discuss	
Temperature	Temperature should be in the region of 36.5–37.4 °C. If cold, warm while assessing heart/respiratory rate and general behaviour. Only re-commence examination when baby is warm and no anomalies found	
Colour	Well perfused? Jaundiced: predisposing factors, does the baby appear well? Conduct appropriate assessment of babies with darker skin tones	
Head	Suture lines/integrity of skull bones Fontanelles: number, size, normal? Facial features: dysmorphia, asymmetry Ears: shape, size	*Head circumference*: tape measure should be placed round widest part of the baby's head with the centimetre edge just above the brow line
Neck/clavicles	Neck: tumours or webbing. Clavicles: fractures or indentations	
Palate	Digital and visual inspection: teeth present? Evidence of tongue tie? Are the soft and hard palate complete?	
Posture/behaviour	Assess tone, good flexion, normal movements and responsiveness to speech, light and touch	
Heart rate	Normal apex beat = 100–160/min	
Respiratory	Normal respiratory rate = 30–60/min. Normal breathing movements with equal chest rise on both sides and no chest recession	
Chest	Normal shape, two nipples equally spaced. Presence of gynaecomastia?	
Abdomen	Normal frontal 'pot-bellied' shape, smooth and no masses visible	
Umbilicus	Correct number of vessels in cord. Correct placement of cord clamp and that it is secure No visible sign of herniation	
Upper limbs	Count number of digits on left and right hands, by slightly separating each one as it is counted Palm creases × 2 – if only 1 crease, is this familial or are there any other dysmorphic features? Check there is nothing hiding in the palms of the hands and for interdigital webbing. Check bone integrity, movement	
Lower limbs	Count number of digits on left and right feet, by slightly separating each one as it is counted, and assess for interdigital webbing. Check for normal plantar creases and long bone integrity Assess for normal movement of legs, signs of talipes (also check the soles of the feet), rocker-bottom shape	
Genitalia	*Male* Check if penis appears normal and no presence of epispadias or hypospadias Epstein's pearl at tip of penis or any part of genitalia? Are both testes descended in a scrotal sac of normal appearance?	*Female* Normal appearance with labia majora slightly oedematous Any sign of vaginal skin tags, overlarge clitoris (female sex characteristics may be difficult to define) or obvious imperforate hymen
Spine	Check the integrity of the spine by placing the baby tummy down over the hand while holding them slightly off the cot bed (with large babies let the baby's knees rest on the cot), which action allows the spinal vertebrae to open slightly. Gently draw a finger smoothly down the spine from the nape of the hair to the coccyx. **Do not** drag the skin with your finger. Check for integrity of the spine and presence of hair tufts, sacral dimple and birth marks. Rotate the baby so that you can view and inspect the side of the baby that until now has been facing away from you	
Eyes	Check that both eyes are present and for normal appearance in terms of shape, size and alignment. During the period after birth the baby is often attentive and can demonstrate the ability to 'fixate'	
Skin	Assess the condition of the skin, noting any sign of trauma. Check for rashes and birth marks, noting size, shape and colour as necessary on a body map – inform the parent(s) that you are doing this and why	
Anus	Note appearance and position of anal opening and if the baby passed meconium in utero or soon after delivery **NOTE:** the anus can only be termed 'patent' if it looks normal and the passage of meconium through the anus has been witnessed	
Urine	Passage of urine should be noted and, if witnessed, whether the steam of urine was smooth, not 'stuttering'	
Neurological	Reflexes, alertness and responsiveness will be assessed as the initial examination of the newborn progresses. All key reflexes should be noted when demonstrated by the baby, for example blinking, ability to suckle, normal hand and feet reflexes etc. (see Chapter 35 regarding neonatal reflexes)	
Weight	Check that scales are calibrated to nought and nothing is touching them. Allow measurement to settle before recording. Inform parent(s), giving both metric and imperial measurements	
Communication	*Parent(s)*: inform of findings, where you are documenting the information and who has access to that information. Answer any queries *Paediatrician*: In the event of finding an anomaly, give full history in terms of relevant family, antenatal and intrapartum history, plus baby's behaviour since birth and the finding of concern	

Physical Examination of the Newborn at a Glance, Second Edition. Dr Lyn Dolby and Denise (Dee) Campbell.
© 2025 John Wiley & Sons Ltd. Published 2025 by John Wiley & Sons Ltd.

The birth of a baby is a significant event in the life of their parent(s). For many parent the minutes after birth are very emotional and include concerns about the baby's condition.

At birth, an immediate concern usually relates to the baby's ability to accomplish the initial changes that are required in order to adapt and survive outside the uterus (see Chapters 10–11 and 13). However, occasionally an abnormality that was not detected during pregnancy presents at or soon after birth. For example, the baby may exhibit signs of a chromosomal abnormality, heart condition or limb abnormality. At these moments the level of professional sensitivity, knowledge and understanding employed will make a significant difference to the parent(s) as the initial impact of the issue of concern sinks in. However, it is paramount that if anomalies are found, these concerns must be expressed to the parent(s) followed by an explanation regarding the action that will be taken.

Most of the babies examined will have no problem adapting to extrauterine life. Therefore, this is a time for the parent(s) to get to know the signs of a healthy baby and what are issues of concern. Parent(s) also need to be informed that their baby is undergoing considerable physiological changes and should not be viewed as a 'miniature adult'. The neonatal period denotes the duration of time when most of the major adaptations to extrauterine life take place. This is why the assessment of neonatal health and well-being usually progresses as follows: the initial examination of the baby at birth, followed by the examination of the newborn within 72 hours of birth and finally the 6 to 8 week infant examination with the GP, unless there is any cause for concern.

Initial examination at birth

Under normal circumstances, this initial examination can be performed within the first hour post birth, after the parent(s) have had time to look at and cuddle their baby. The examination should be performed where it can be easily witnessed by the parent(s) and the lighting is good, preferably in natural daylight. Hands should be washed and dried prior to the examination and everything required should be close at hand (e.g. scales and baby clothes). The examination should be performed quickly and comprehensively, only uncovering the part of the baby to be examined and re-covering them as soon as practicable in order to assist them in maintaining normal body temperature during a time when this has not yet stabilised.

The initial examination should always include the following points:
• Commence with an exploration of the maternal and neonatal notes, assessing for relevant predisposing factors that may indicate the possibility of compromise to newborn health. Any issue arising during the antenatal period and/or correspondence from the paediatric team or other professional expert or institution should also be taken into account and the parent(s)' knowledge of it ascertained.
• Parent(s) should always be informed about what the examination process entails and their ability to understand what is being said needs to be determined. An interpreting or translation service may be required.
• Prior to commencing the examination, parental consent must always be obtained. Inform the parent(s) that the baby may cry but that this is usually because of the stimuli of cooler temperature, light, touch and sound.
• Parent(s) should be asked for their impression of their baby's health and if they have any concerns, which may include issues that have arisen during the antenatal period.

• The baby should be examined in full view of at least one of the parents.
• The examination should follow a systematic process in order not to miss any aspect of the examination (Table 24.1).
• The parent(s) should be fully informed of the findings of the examination, their baby's abilities as a newborn, for example the ability to fixate with the eyes, and the neurological reflexes that are present and why.
• Specific newborn care practices should be discussed if they relate to the findings of the examination, culture and/or religion. For example, the parent(s) may come from a culture that frequently swaddles their babies, or an epispadias has been noted on examination but it may be common in the parent(s)' religion or culture to circumcise baby boys (see Chapter 51).

After the examination

Any anomaly must be appropriately and accurately recorded and referral sought if required. In the event of birth marks it is particularly important to draw a body diagram to depict position, colour and size, especially if the birth mark could be confused with non-accidental injury (see Chapters 36 and 37). Parent(s) must be informed that this record has been made and why.

If this has not already been performed, the baby should be weighed naked. Attention should be paid at this stage to making sure that the scales are properly calibrated, that the examiner does not accidently lean on the scales or that part of the scale is not touching anything else that may cause an inaccurate reading to be taken.

Administration of vitamin K should already have been discussed with the parent(s), but this should be broached again as they need to be clear what vitamin K is administered for, where and how it is administered. They may decide in the light of antenatal and intrapartum factors that it is not required, which should be recorded. The options in relation to method and routes of administration do depend in part on what is available in differing parts of the country. If oral vitamin K is chosen, parent(s) need to know about follow-up administration.

Finally, the baby should be dressed and a hat put on their head. There may still be some residual dampness within the hair and a hat assists in keeping the baby warm while their temperature control mechanisms stabilise. The hat should be removed after approximately six hours in the healthy term baby, who should by this point be able to maintain their own temperature reasonably well, and this also introduces the fact that a hat should not be required indoors.

The examiner must role model good behaviour from the start. For example, the baby should be placed in the cot on their back, with the bed clothing placed appropriately to assist in safe sleeping practices (see Chapter 6).

Returning the baby to the parent(s) may only necessitate placing a nappy on the baby if the mother wishes to hold her baby skin to skin. This position will reduce stress on the baby, settling and calming their vital signs and encouraging them to root and breastfeed. This is a period of time for the parent(s) to be left to bond, hydrate and have some light refreshment while the examination is documented.

All documentation should be fully completed, including any discussions with the paediatrician if required, the weight of the baby, any parental concerns and their wishes regarding method of infant feeding. If vitamin K has been administered, parental consent, the dose, batch number and how/where administered should be clearly recorded.

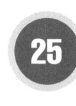

25 Daily examination of the newborn: overview

Table 25.1 Key areas of assessment in the daily examination of the newborn.

Aspect	Observe and assess the following elements	
Predisposing factors	Investigate *Recorded history*: family, antenatal, intrapartum and maternal/neonatal progress or concerns since birth *Ask parent(s)*: for information on any concerns about their baby that they wish to discuss	
Temperature	Temperature should be within the realms of normality (36.5–37.4 °C). Unless the baby has previously been noted to have been hypothermic or feels cooler than expected to the touch (on upper chest and between scapulae), there should be no need to take their temperature. However, if they are cold, warm while assessing heart/respiratory rate and general behaviour. Only recommence examination when baby is warm and no anomalies found	
Colour	Well perfused Jaundiced: predisposing factors, yellowing of the skin in relation to age post birth, does the baby appear well? Conduct appropriate assessment of babies with darker skin tones	
Head	Status of moulding, bruising or other trauma arising from delivery Only measure the head circumference if there is any query concerning the measurement taken at birth or any other factors that can impact on head size	
Neck/clavicles	Neck: observe for signs of chafing, soreness etc. Clavicles: observe for bruising, changes to visual appearance	
Palate/mouth	Palate: only review if there are signs of concern (e.g. milk often comes out of the baby's nose) Mouth: well perfused, presence of milk residue only, no signs of thrush, bleeding or soreness	
Posture/behaviour	Assess tone, flexion, normal movements and responsiveness to speech, light and touch	
Heart rate	Apex beat should still reflect normality (100–160/min), but only reassess if there are signs of concern	
Respiratory	Respiratory rate should still reflect normality (30–60/min), but only reassess if there are signs of concern	
Umbilicus	Depending on the number of days since birth, check if clamp secure, no signs of flaring or odour and that normal process of separation is occurring	
Upper limbs	Assess that general movement is within the range of normality	
Lower limbs	Assess that general movement is within the range of normality	
Genitalia/excretion	*Male* Assess for signs of soreness or infection, bruising or condition of hydrocoele if present Is there a good urine flow on micturition?	*Female* Assess for signs of soreness or infection Signs of mucous, pseudo-menstruation?
	Note if the baby has passed urine or meconium and how often – link to feeding ability Is the anus patent? The passage of nitrates may be seen as a small orange patch in the nappy Any sign of nappy rash?	
Eyes	Assess if eyes are 'sticky' or if there are signs of infection	
Skin – general	Assess the condition of the skin, noting any sign of trauma. Check for rashes and birth marks, noting size, shape and colour as necessary	
Neurological	Reflexes will be assessed when the examination of the newborn is performed, but the ability of the baby to blink, grasp a finger, suckle and demonstrate a Moro reflex should be observed (see Chapter 35 regarding neonatal reflexes) Any odd or abnormal movements should be observed, documented (with any related findings) and a referral made to the paediatric team Assess alertness and responsiveness	
Feeding	Note method of feeding, frequency (relate to post-birth age) and link with quantity of excretion Is baby waking for feeds, settling after feeds? Is feeding support required? Investigate if parent(s) know where to obtain help with feeding	
Communication	Inform parent(s) of the daily examination findings and any further information they need at the present post-birth age Maternal/parental interactions with their newborn baby should be observed in a sensitive manner Parental fears or concerns should be listened to and not dismissed Time spent with a parent is never time wasted	

The first 3–4 weeks after a baby's birth constitute a significant period of learning not only for parents but also the baby. Most babies have managed to accomplish the initial adaptations to extrauterine life, but their continuing progress and development will need careful observation during the neonatal period. It is for this reason that the daily examination is an important part of neonatal care, as it is not only a time of observation and reassessment of the baby's progress, but also a time of sharing information with the parent(s) in relation to their baby's physiological status and their ability to interact with and react to the people and the world around them. This is also a time when parent(s) should be reminded that their baby is not a miniature adult and that they are undergoing considerable physiological changes. However, many NHS Trusts operate a reduced service of post-natal care that in

Physical Examination of the Newborn at a Glance, Second Edition. Dr Lyn Dolby and Denise (Dee) Campbell.
© 2025 John Wiley & Sons Ltd. Published 2025 by John Wiley & Sons Ltd.

some instances includes telephone conversations instead of face-to-face meetings. Each qualified midwife must bear in mind the requirements of their professionalism in relation to The Code (NMC, 2018) and the Standards of Proficiency for Midwives (NMC, 2019). A blanket approach to care will not provide a high standard of care to all parents and their newborns, since for example those who need greater support or assessment such as babies with darker skin tones need visual observation to detect signs of jaundice. Therefore, each midwife will need to work with managers to ensure that the parents and babies in their catchment area have access to the care required, which can in itself reduce costs relating to re-admission and increased treatment requirements occurring due to less than timely recognition of the changing status of mother or baby.

Daily examination of the newborn

Under normal circumstances, this daily examination should be performed when it is convenient for both mother and baby. Preferably, the baby should be in the 'quiet, alert' state of consciousness if their ongoing development of health and well-being is to be comprehensively assessed. As with the initial examination, the baby should be examined where they can be easily witnessed by the parent(s) and the lighting is good, ideally in natural daylight. Hands should be washed and dried prior to the examination and everything required should be close at hand (e.g. clean nappy, bowl of warm water etc.).

Always assess the baby's temperature first, particularly if this is the first daily examination or if the parent(s) have voiced concerns about their baby's behaviour. If the baby is over 6 hours old and still has a hat on indoors, this can be removed and the parent(s) informed that babies only need hats if outdoors (warm hat for cold conditions and sunhat at other times). If the baby has previously been noted to have had a low temperature, use a suitable means of temperature measurement so that an accurate assessment can be made. If the baby's temperature is below normal thresholds, then they should not be undressed further (unless skin to skin is advocated) and a hat should be placed on the baby's head. An investigation should be commenced to determine why the baby became cold and appropriate management undertaken.

The daily examination should always include the following key points:
• Commence with an exploration of the available records in order to determine if any changes have occurred since birth. If the examiner is seeing this baby for the first time, they should check for relevant predisposing factors that may indicate the possibility of compromise to newborn health. Any issue arising during the antenatal period and/or correspondence from the paediatric team or other professional expert or institution should also be taken into account and the parent(s)' knowledge of this ascertained.
• Discuss with the parent(s) any concerns they may have and, as with the initial examination, inform them what the examination process entails. Their understanding of what is said and the terms used should be assessed.
• Parental consent for the examination must always be obtained.
• The baby should be examined in full view of the parent(s).
• The examination should follow a systematic process in order not to miss any aspect of the process (see Table 25.1 for key areas).
• Give a comprehensive explanation of the findings of the examination.
• If appropriate, the parent(s) should be informed about why jaundice may occur, which is particularly important if the baby has obvious signs of trauma or bruising from delivery or any risk factors for pathological jaundice.
• Feeding progress should be discussed and support given with feeding and/or observe the baby when feeding if required.

• Skin care and care of the umbilicus are important, as many parents are unaware how thin the baby's skin layer is, or how the chemicals within any preparation used on the skin can be partly absorbed. They need to know how detrimental urine and faeces can be to the skin, how to avoid soreness and chafing. Information about any particular skin preparations that can be used that have little impact on the physiology of the skin should be discussed. The practitioner should be fully conversant with the contemporary literature in order to accomplish this effectively.
• This is a good time to discuss the baby's abilities and to point out signs of good health, such as how alert the baby is, their attentiveness, how to recognise changes in colour or perfusion, how to check the baby is warm enough (place the back of the hand on the baby's chest or between the scapulae) or to draw attention to normal posture, behaviour and muscle tone.
• As with the initial examination, specific newborn care practices should be discussed. It may only be during the daily examination that particular care practices relating to culture, tradition or religion come to light. For example, the parent(s) may come from a culture that frequently swaddles their babies, which can reduce the development of the hip joint and cause over-heating.

After the examination

Any adverse findings must be appropriately and accurately recorded and referral sought if required. In the event of skin changes, it should be determined whether these are caused by normal physiology, such as in the case of erythema toxicum neonatorum, or whether they are of a nature that is more concerning, such as an odd subtle birthmark or the presence of pustular spots that may be indicative of infection.

If the baby was found to have been placed on their side or stomach to sleep, the practitioner needs to discuss the key aspects of safer sleeping in a sensitive but informed manner (see Chapter 6). This may also mean that the sleeping position of the baby in the cot is demonstrated so that the parent(s) have not only a verbal image but a visual one too.

A comprehensive record of the examination must be completed, including an indication of how feeding is progressing and the quantity of 'wet' and 'dirty' nappies (and if the consistency is changing). Any parental concerns should be recorded and information given in response and/or actions taken.

Maternal well-being

The daily examination is not just about reviewing the baby's health and well-being, it is also a time when maternal or parental reactions to their newborn baby can be quietly observed. The 'bonding' process between parent and baby is not always an easy one and not all parents love their child the instant they are born. For some, these early days are a period of change, uncertainty and concern about their own abilities as parents. For others, there may be various issues that are impacting on their ability to care for themselves, let alone this newborn baby. The effect of a parent's mental health on themselves, the baby and the wider family can be considerable (RCOG, 2017; NICE, 2023b; Maternal Mental Health Alliance, 2023).

The daily examination of the newborn may at first appear to be solely focused on the baby, but observing the interaction between baby and parent(s) is just as important in relation to health and well-being. Practitioners should be conversant with the available guidance and policies and be aware of any shortcomings within their own knowledge base if those parents who need extra assistance are to be recognised early and provided with appropriate care. Remember, the time you spend with parents is *never* time wasted.

26 Newborn blood spot screening

Table 26.1 Conditions that are part of the newborn blood spot screening programme.

Condition	Details	Management
Sickle cell disease (SCD)	An autosomal recessive inherited condition that affects haemoglobin Incidence: 1 in 2200 babies in England 1 in 74 carriers are detected Present at birth, but signs of SCD may not appear until after 4 months of age Babies with this condition will need specialist care throughout their lives If untreated: high risk of death or complications from treatable infections, severe acute anaemia and stroke in the first few years of life It can cause attacks of very severe pain, life-threatening infections and anaemia Ongoing parental support is required	Early treatment recommended, including childhood immunisations Oral penicillin and Prevenar vaccine before 3 months of age to reduce the chance of serious illness **Note:** babies with beta-thalassaemia major – the most serious form of thalassaemia – will generally be detected by screening, but carriers are not detected
Cystic fibrosis (CF)	An autosomal recessive inherited condition affecting the digestive system and lungs Incidence: 1 in 2500 in the United Kingdom Symptoms usually begin in early childhood, with poor weight gain and frequent chest infections If untreated: leads to lung damage, poor growth and development Survival: mean age 41	Early treatment – high-energy diet, medication and regular physiotherapy commencing by 30 days of age **Note:** some babies require a second blood sample for further testing on day 21 Not all carriers will be identified
Congenital hypothyroidism (CHT)	There are a number of causes for hypothyroidism, but it is not usually inherited Incidence: 1 in 3000 babies in the United Kingdom A condition in which insufficient thyroxine is produced Babies do not have any problems at birth, but if left untreated permanent physical and mental disability will develop	Treatment commences with thyroxine therapy by 21 days of age to allow normal development

Table 26.2 Inherited metabolic diseases (IMDs) that are part of the newborn blood spot screening programme.

The following six IMDs are all autosomal recessive inherited metabolic diseases, which cause the problems noted.	
Phenylketonuria (PKU)	Impact: difficulty with breaking down the phenylalanine amino acid Incidence: 1 in 10,000 in the United Kingdom
Medium-chain acyl-coenzyme A dehydrogenase deficiency (MCADD)	Impact: difficulty with breaking down fat Incidence: 1 in 10,000 in the United Kingdom
Maple syrup urine disease (MSUD)	Impact: difficulty with breaking down leucine, isoleucine and valine amino acids Incidence: 1 in 116,000 in the United Kingdom
Isovaleric acidaemia (IVA)	Impact: difficulty with breaking down the leucine amino acid Incidence: 1 in 155,000 in the European Union
Glutaric aciduria type 1 (GA1)	Impact: difficulty with breaking down lysine and tryptophan amino acids Incidence: 1 in 110,000 in the European Union
Homocystinuria (pyridoxine unresponsive) (HCU)	Impact: prevents the breakdown of the homocysteine amino acid Incidence: 1 in 144,000 in United Kingdom

Table 26.3 Metabolic condition recommended for inclusion in the newborn blood spot screening (NBS) programme.

Tyrosinaemia type 1	Rare metabolic disorder of which there are three types (type 1 is the least rare and all are inherited in a recessive pattern) Each type is caused by a lack of a functional copy of a different key enzyme in the process by which tyrosine is broken down The body is unable to breakdown amino acid tyrosine (a component part of the proteins in the body and food) Children with type 1 tyrosinaemia usually show symptoms at approx. 6 months of age, by which time liver damage has already occurred
Impact	Liver problems are common in type 1: as the missing enzyme is primarily related to liver cells, tyrosine is partially but not completely broken down. This allows molecules (e.g. succinylacetate), to accumulate within the cells, causing toxicity. Resulting damage can lead to liver failure, increased risk of liver cancer, kidney dysfunction, learning difficulties and neurological crisis (e.g. limb pain, vomiting and seizures)
Management	Special diet, reducing the intake of the amino acids tyrosine and phenylalanine – symptoms can be eased or negated Previously liver transplant was the only option for many patients, but more recently a drug treatment called nitisinone has been developed that prevents the formation of toxic elements
At present there is ongoing research to review other conditions that can be included within the NBS screening programme and therefore it is essential to review the content and new information as it is entered onto the NBS website.	

Physical Examination of the Newborn at a Glance, Second Edition. Dr Lyn Dolby and Denise (Dee) Campbell.
© 2025 John Wiley & Sons Ltd. Published 2025 by John Wiley & Sons Ltd.

Table 26.4 Ongoing research: severe combined immunodeficiency (SCID).

SCID has impacts on the immune system, making it hard for a baby to fight off infections such as meningitis and pneumonia. Both infections can be life-threatening and approximately 14 babies born each year in England have SCID
Present research
In some areas of England, testing for SCID is being offered as part of the newborn blood spot test. This is part of ongoing research to assist the screening committee to decide whether testing for SCID should be offered to all babies in England

The UK National Screening Committee (NSC) issues guidance, support and training on various conditions that can affect the health of individuals. For some conditions a national programme of screening has been established in order to detect these conditions early, provide pre-emptive treatment and reduce the cost to the health of the individual as well as the financial costs incurred for later recognition and treatment. Therefore, as with any widespread screening programme, the cost of screening has to be balanced with the acceptability of the screening rationale and method, the impact on the health of the individual, the prevalence of the condition and the ability to treat or manage the condition effectively.

Newborn blood spot (NBS) screening is one of the areas that is covered by a national screening programme. It enables identification of babies who may have rare but serious conditions. The number of babies affected may be small, but early detection, referral and treatment can help to improve their health and prevent severe disability or, in some cases, death.

The UK NSC recommends that all babies are offered screening and at present this consists of the conditions highlighted in Table 26.1 and also six inherited metabolic diseases (IMDs) (Table 26.2). The UK NSC has also recommended inclusion of testing for tyrosinaemia type 1 within the NBS (see Table 26.3). Ongoing research is being conducted to determine the feasibility of testing all babies for severe combined immunodeficiency (SCID) – see Table 26.4 for further information.

Prior to or during the antenatal booking session, a copy of the booklet 'Screening tests for you and your baby' should be given to all who are pregnant. This is also a good time to ascertain from the parent(s) if there is a family history of any of the IMDs so that early screening can be offered if appropriate. For those whose first language is not English, translated versions of the information booklet are available (https://www.gov.uk/government/publications/screening-tests-for-you-and-your-baby).

It is important to offer NBS screening to all parents and to check that those who have just moved into the area with a newborn baby have not missed out on the opportunity to have their baby screened. As with any procedure, parents need comprehensive information about the screening programme, what it tests for, how the sampling is conducted and the possible outcomes if their baby tests positive for any of the conditions.

As NBS screening usually takes place on day 5 post birth (day of birth = day 0), NBS screening should ideally be discussed again at least 24 hours prior to the procedure. This gives parents the opportunity to think about the information discussed and engage with the related website in order to decide whether they wish to give their consent. When verbal consent to NBS screening has been given, it should be clearly recorded as 'consent given' in the NHS Trust maternal/neonatal record and/or electronic record and the PCHR.

Parental consent to any research linked to the NBS screening programme should also be ascertained and they should be informed that they can find further information on https://www.nhs.uk/Conditions/pregnancy-and-baby/Pages/newborn-blood-spot-cards.aspx. If a parent does not wish to be contacted about future research in relation to their baby's sample, they will need to know and see evidence that the words 'No research contact' have been recorded clearly on the blood spot card. However, parents do need to be aware that patient-identifiable information may be stored by the NHS Sickle Cell and Thalassaemia Screening Programme. The information relating to this is available online at https://www.gov.uk/government/publications/sickle-cell-and-thalassaemia-screening-newborn-outcomes-system/sct-newborn-outcomes-system-overview.

Parents can decline screening for one or more of the conditions in Table 26.1 – sickle cell disease (SCD), cystic fibrosis (CF) and congenital hypothyroidism (CHT) – but the six IMDs (Table 26.2) can only be declined as a group. In this instance a clear record should be made in the NHS Trust maternal/neonatal record and/or electronic record and the PCHR. This must state clearly which test is being declined and if possible the rationale for the parent(s)' decision. When NBS screening is declined for only one or some of the conditions, the blood spot card should be completed and marked 'Decline – XX' (where XX is the condition(s) that has been declined) and add the rationale if given.

In the event that consent is declined for NBS screening per se, the records should clearly state this decision and the rationale if possible. The blood spot card should also be completed, but this time it should be marked 'Decline – all conditions' and the rationale given if available prior to sending it to the laboratory. Local procedures should be followed in relation to informing the Child Health Records Department, the GP, the health visitor and the NBS lead midwife/manager. A separate letter will also be sent to the parent(s), but they should also be informed verbally who they can contact if they change their mind, would like to discuss any aspect of the screening process or require further information. All of this will need to be recorded in the PCHR.

The sampling process

For the purpose of NBS screening, the day of birth is counted as day 0. The blood spot sample should be taken on day 5 for all babies, but in exceptional circumstances the sample may be taken between days 5 and 8 or may need to be repeated. For example, the baby may have been born prematurely or has recently had a blood transfusion that can affect the test results.

Public Health England produced a guideline for NBS sampling in 2016, which was further updated in 2021 and is available at https://www.gov.uk/government/publications/newborn-blood-spot-screening-sampling-guidelines. All students and practitioners who are involved in NBS screening must be fully conversant with the content of this guideline to enable them to observe best practice in terms of sampling to reduce the number of repeat results caused by poor sampling. There is also an elearning NBS module available when logged into the elfh hub: https://www.elfh.org.uk/programmes/nhsscreeningprogrammes/#:~:text=The%20NHS%20Newborn%20Blood%20Spot,sickle%20cell%20disease%20(SCD).

27 Hearing screening

Figure 27.1 Flowchart showing the screening process.

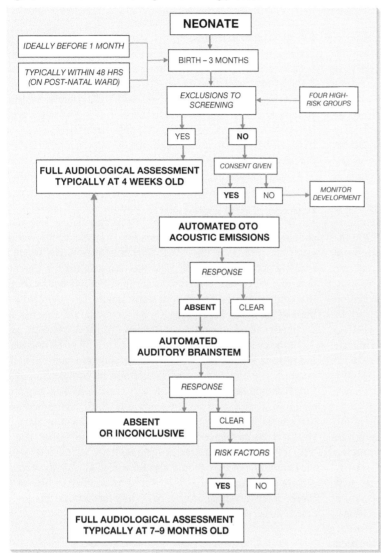

Figure 27.2 Automated otoacoustic emissions testing (AOAE).
Source: Donald Trung Quoc Don/Wikimedia Commons/CC BY SA 4.0.

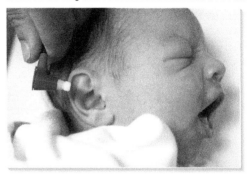

Figure 27.3 Automated auditory brainstem response (AABR) testing.
Source: Dean Johnson/Flickr/CC BY 2.0.

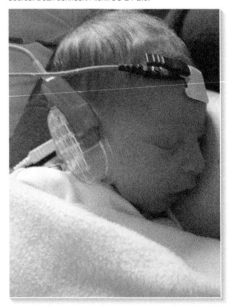

Physical Examination of the Newborn at a Glance, Second Edition. Dr Lyn Dolby and Denise (Dee) Campbell.
© 2025 John Wiley & Sons Ltd. Published 2025 by John Wiley & Sons Ltd.

Early screening for full or partial deafness reduces many long-term health issues and the associated health costs. Detection of a problem with appropriate management improves intellectual, social, psychological and communication outcomes. Prior to the routine early neonatal screening programmes, only those considered high risk were screened and as many as 50% of those with full or partial deafness were missed. The problems were often not identified until they became clinically apparent. Figure 27.1 shows a flow chart for the screening process that is expanded on in what follows.

Exclusions (PHE, 2022)

Babies are excluded if they are less than 34 weeks or over 3 months (corrected age). Additionally, there are four high-risk groups so likely to have partial or full hearing loss that a routine newborn screening test should not be carried out. Instead a **full audiological referral** at 4 weeks is required. The four high-risk groups are babies with:
- Microtia (under-developed pinna) and external ear canal atresia.
- Neonatal bacterial meningitis or meningococcal septicaemia.
- Programmable ventriculo-peritoneal (PVP) shunts in place.
- Confirmed congenital cytomegalovirus (referred before 4 weeks).

Informed choice

Leaflets are available in various languages and discussions with healthcare professionals can clarify any concerns parents may have. Information should be shared about:
- Procedures involved in screening.
- Painless nature of the various tests involved.
- Follow-up processes that may be required.
- Advantages of early detection.
- Only known risk – the possibility of a false positive and the associated anxieties.
- Why false positives may occur: for example uncooperative, distressed newborn; background noise or interference; faulty equipment; or temporary deafness/blocking of the auditory canal.

Referral for screening (PHE, 2019)

Most commonly hearing screening takes place on the post-natal ward prior to discharge and within 48 hours of birth. It is performed by trained audiologists who make daily visits to the ward. In some circumstances, such as following a home birth or over a bank holiday, referral may be required to an alternative designated professional for the tests. This may be to an individual (such as a health visitor) or to an audiology clinic. It should ideally be within a month of the birth for a healthy term newborn, but can be still carried out up to three months after delivery. For a premature infant the optimum time is calculated based on the expected date of delivery.

Screening tests used

Automated otoacoustic emissions (AOAE) (Figure 27.2)

This can be used from a few hours after birth. It is painless and takes only a few minutes. The parent/carer can stay with the newborn throughout. A soft earpiece is inserted into the ear and clicking noises are played through it. A normal cochlea will then emit a responsive reaction, detected by the test equipment. A clear response from both ears is reassuring of no early-onset deafness. This test has the advantage of a non-invasive, speedy result, but is associated with higher false-negative rates. In the absence of a clear response, the second screening test is used.

Automated auditory brainstem response (AABR) (Figure 27.3)

This test requires a restful, preferably sleeping, newborn and a suitably quiet environment away from other noisy stimuli. Parents or carers can stay with the newborn and can be reassured that the test is painless and takes only 5–15 minutes. This test examines the full pathway for hearing, going beyond the cochlea to monitor brainstem responses. It involves sounds being played through headphones or occasionally ear probes may be used. Sensors are typically attached on the forehead and shoulder but sometimes also the nape of the neck. Before the sensors are put in place the skin will be cleaned with special wipes and allowed to dry, then a conductive gel is applied and the sensors attached with sticky pads.

Professional responsibilities

The professional carrying out the physical examination of the newborn must verify that one of the following has occurred.
- Screening has been discussed but consent was withheld.
  - A non-judgemental approach is taken and everything documented.
  - GP and health visitor are made aware.
  - The parent/carer has been encouraged to monitor ongoing progress using the developmental checklists and to notify any concerns.
- Screening has been completed with a clear response in both ears.
  - Everything has been appropriately documented.
  - Possibility of late-onset deafness has been discussed and the parent/carer has been encouraged to monitor ongoing progress using the developmental checklists and to notify any concerns.
  - A clear response letter has been given to the parent/carer.
  - Risk factors and follow-up needs have been considered.
- Screening has been completed with an inconclusive or non-clear response in one or both ears.
  - Everything has been appropriately documented.
  - A follow-up hearing specialist/audiology clinic appointment has been arranged for four weeks after the initial tests.
  - The carer has been given an explanation and encouraged to monitor their newborn's progress using the developmental checklists.

Targeted post-routine screening (PHE, 2019)

Even when the AABR screening test is clear for both ears, the presence of risk factors requires a referral for audiological and behavioural assessment at 7–8 months old. Risk factors include:
- Congenital infections (e.g. rubella, toxoplasmosis).
- Syndromes associated with hearing loss (e.g. trisomy 21).
- Cranio-facial abnormalities (including cleft palate).
- Parental/professional developmental concerns or family history.
- Admissions to an SCBU or NICU for longer than 48 hours.
- Ototoxic drug received (e.g. aminoglycosides, gentamicin).
- Medical conditions linked to hearing loss (e.g. temporal bone fracture, cytomegalovirus, severe unconjugated hyperbilirubinaemia, bacterial meningitis, meningococcal septicaemia).

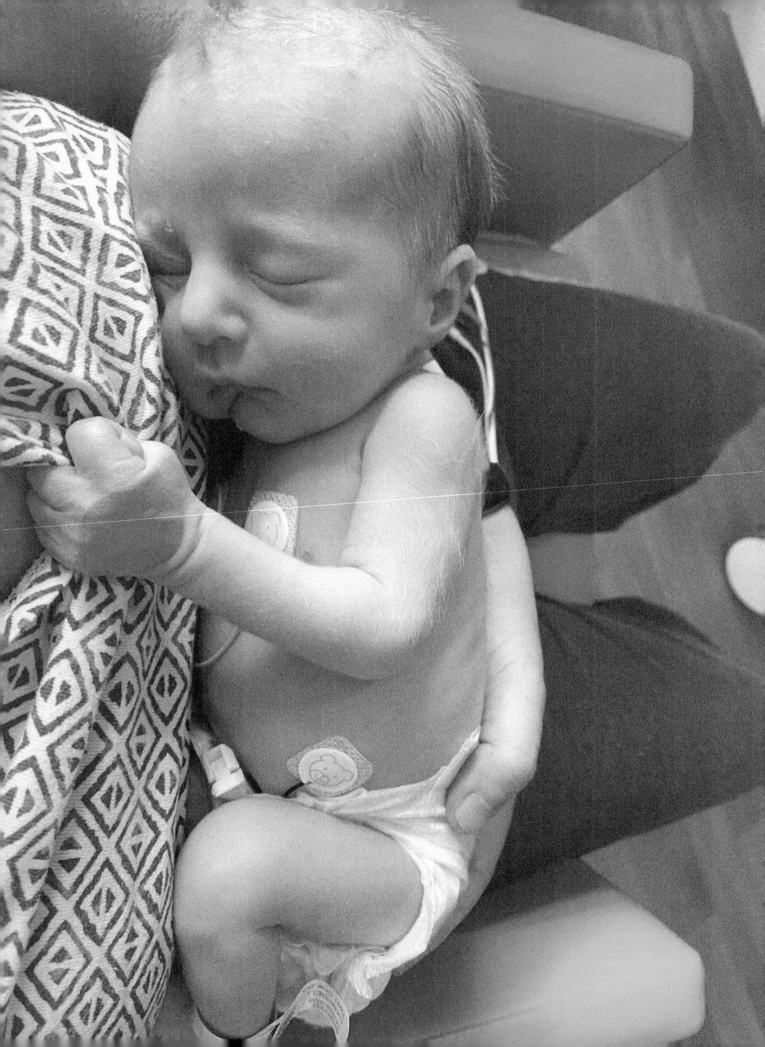

Prior to the physical examination

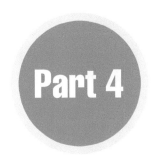

Part 4

Chapters

28 Preparing to examine

Figure 28.1 Neonatal stethoscope head (chest piece).

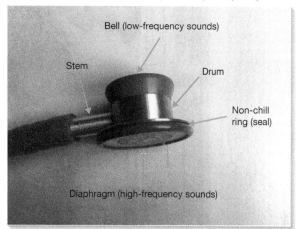

Bell (low-frequency sounds)

Stem

Drum

Non-chill ring (seal)

Diaphragm (high-frequency sounds)

Figure 28.2 Neonatal stethoscope.

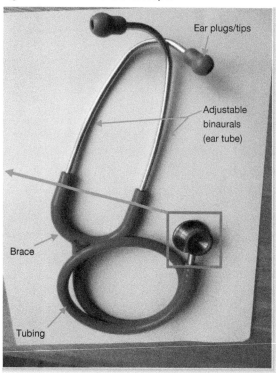

Ear plugs/tips

Adjustable binaurals (ear tube)

Brace

Tubing

Figure 28.3 Pocket ophthalmoscope (side view).

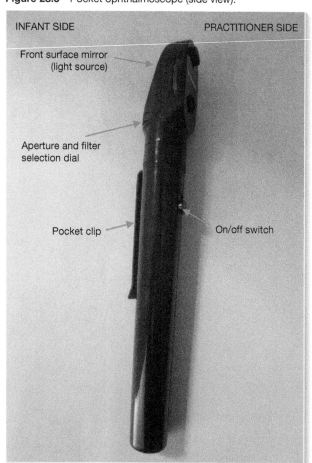

INFANT SIDE

PRACTITIONER SIDE

Front surface mirror (light source)

Aperture and filter selection dial

Pocket clip

On/off switch

Figure 28.4 Ophthalmoscope head (practitioner side).

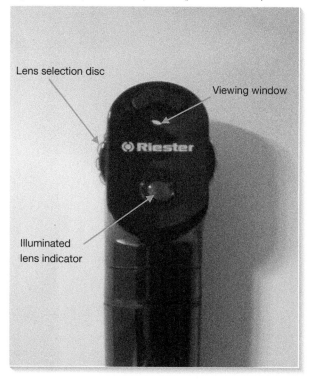

Lens selection disc

Viewing window

Riester

Illuminated lens indicator

Physical Examination of the Newborn at a Glance, Second Edition. Dr Lyn Dolby and Denise (Dee) Campbell.
© 2025 John Wiley & Sons Ltd. Published 2025 by John Wiley & Sons Ltd.

Predicting concerns

The physical examination commences with the review of all relevant histories, to inform the examination and its outcome. All information gleaned from the records should be viewed as a screening tool that informs the practitioner about the infant's higher or lower probability of risk. While it is possible that a competent practitioner would identify any physical abnormalities even without this additional information, this knowledge enables an individualised approach to risk and greater sensitivity to the specific concerns of the family.

History alone can alert the practitioner to further screening and diagnostic care required (aligned to the local policies and protocols), for instance a concerning antenatal scan, breech presentation or difficult delivery. The practitioner will be looking for any possible neonatal impact from maternal health issues (e.g. infection, diabetes and anaemia) or surgical intervention (e.g. forceps or ventouse delivery). Socio-demographics such as age, obesity and smoking habits will guide health promotion discussions. The health of siblings may also have an impact, for example hearing impairment or an identified child protection concern (a child protection plan may already be in place for this neonate). A combination of prior history and the current examination will guide additional screening and referrals, including to whom, when, where and how these referrals should be made.

Awareness of a client's history is part of the professional role. This must be treated with sensitivity on a 'need to know' basis to support client confidentiality. Analysis of the information is from the perspective of how aspects may directly, or indirectly, impact on the current health and future development of the infant.

Parental concerns

Specific screening tests will already have been performed antenatally and the results will impact the neonatal examination. This is not only linked to occasions when screening has identified a higher-risk situation, but also because the discussions around reliability of screening tests will have introduced awareness for the family around false-positive and false-negative results. Sadly, they may have been left with increased awareness of neonatal health risks but without a complete guarantee that their baby is not affected. Diagnostic tests may also have been carried out or may have been decided against because of their own inherent health risks for the fetus.

The practitioner is expected to have some knowledge of how genetic and inherent conditions or physical abnormalities may occur to enable informed discussions. Seek advice and increase awareness about these before approaching the family. Speak with the midwife providing daily care to ensure you have the most up-to-date information.

Parents may consider the physical examination as a way they can be finally reassured about the health of their baby. The practitioner should be aware of tests that have been carried out and their results before entering a conversation with the family. It is essential that the limitations of the examination are clearly explained. Reassurances may follow the examination and greater clarity may be possible around identified concerns, but the examination is itself only a screening tool with its own limitations. The fetal transition to newborn life is still ongoing at 72 hours, so the examination can only relate to the specific moment in time that it takes place and this is particularly true for the heart.

Collect equipment

- **Tape measure** – disposable, flexible, clearly printed in centimetres and non-stretchable.
- **Stethoscope** (Figures 28.1 and 28.2) – a specific paediatric one (some adult-size cardiac stethoscopes can be fitted with a paediatric use diaphragm). The stethoscope must be clean and maintained in good working order with no signs of damage related to the diaphragm, ear pieces or tubing; a dual head able to rotate 180° without resistance; and working seals to prevent air loss (air escape noises can affect hearing heart sounds and murmurs).
- **Ophthalmoscope** (Figures 28.3 and 28.4) – a direct vision one. The ophthalmoscope required for viewing the red reflex can be a basic design, but must be clean, maintained in good working order and provide a good light source, with a large round aperture and a means to focus the reflected image.
- **Documentation** – the notes should have already been reviewed for risk factors, but the paediatric and post-natal aspects are needed to record examination results. The PCHR, also known as the 'red book', is provided for every newborn baby to maintain an ongoing health and development record. This includes a page for the neonatal physical examination results.
- **Clean nappy and changing equipment** – to be used as required to facilitate clear viewing of the genitalia, buttocks and upper thigh; allow accurate examination of femoral pulses; and assess for developmental dysplasia of the hips (DDH).

Consider the environment

The environment for the examination can affect the neonate, family and practitioner as well as impacting on the ability to communicate.
- **Privacy** – away from the hearing of others to allow opportunity for honest and sensitive communications.
- **Warmth** – the infant is undressed and is either uncovered or semi-covered during the examination, so a warm room is needed to help the balance of the baby's immature thermoregulation system. An item of clothing or a blanket should be available to cover areas of the baby that have already been fully visualised and examined or between elements of the examination, perhaps when communicating with the parent(s).
- **Lighting** – this must provide the opportunity to see the infant's skin colour in good natural lighting. Additionally, the opportunity to reduce lighting can help calm an infant and enable the red reflex examination.
- **Infant position** – safe, on a firm mattress and at a suitable height for good access.
- **Access to handwashing facilities** – handwashing is required before and after the examination. It must occur after any nappy changing procedure or contact with vomit, urine or stool. This is a standard precaution within infection control.

Some practitioners perform the examination on a resuscitaire within a nursery. This can be an appropriate environment with parental consent, but may require reassurances around the equipment present. It also requires comfortable seating for the parent(s), who should not be excluded.

29 Infection control

Figure 29.1 The stages of hand washing or gel application.
Source: Adapted from Thomas RK (2015). Practical medical procedures at a glance. John Wiley & Sons. It is currently on page 14.

Wet hands and apply soap or apply hand gel to dry hands	Rub hands palm to palm	Continue palm to palm but now interlace fingers as you rub

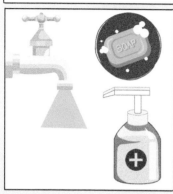 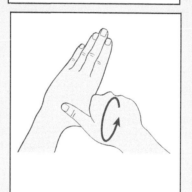 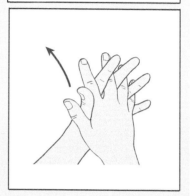

Rub palm to back of hand with fingers interlaced – repeat to second hand	Interlock fingers within palms and rub to clean backs of fingers	Clasp left thumb in palm and rotate then do opposite thumb

Rub tips of fingers and thumb against palm; swap hands and repeat	Rub each wrist with opposite hand	Rinse well. Dry thoroughly with single-use towels. Moisturise

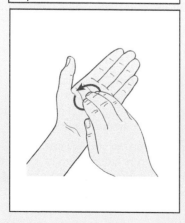 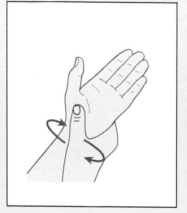 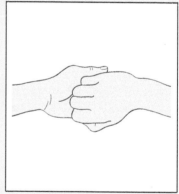 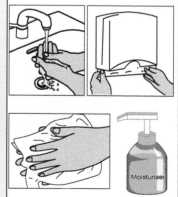

This chapter considers the infection control responsibilities of the professional performing the physical examination. They must:

- Ensure that they do not introduce infection.
- Identify infection already affecting the infant.
- Initiate appropriate treatment of any infection.
- Control against the spread of infection.
- Participate in the education of parents.
- Lead by example.

Infection risks

Healthcare-acquired infections (HAIs) are infections that occur when care is provided by health professionals, in a hospital or the community. The risk of HAI in an acute care hospital is 7% across high-income countries, rising to as high as 15% in low- or middle-income countries, with 1 in every 10 of those affected dying (WHO, 2022). The WHO (2021) figures for Europe confirm that there are now nearly 9 million recorded HAI events across Europe. Significantly, the WHO (2022) also identified that newborns were among those at greatest risk due to the following:

- Increased levels of bacteria within hospital environments – air borne as well as carried by staff and equipment.
- Lowered resistance.
- Exposure as a fetus, e.g. prolonged rupture of membranes, fetal blood sampling.
- Increased maternal infection risk due to e.g. anaemia, operative delivery.
- Close proximity within maternity wards increasing risk of spread.
- Sharing of equipment.
- Warm atmosphere allowing bacteria to multiply.
- High visitor numbers.
- High handling numbers.
- Invasive procedures, e.g. capillary blood sampling.
- Increased likelihood of body fluid exposure.

Infection prevention

Infection prevention is enhanced through an understanding of how infection may be transmitted during the physical examination and the standard precautions that reduce this occurrence. The value of decontamination during hand hygiene was first appreciated by Ignaz Semmelweis in 1847. He was investigating considerably higher levels of puerperal fever in a clinic visited by medical students compared to one run solely by midwives. His breakthrough came when a colleague was accidentally cut by a medical student's scalpel during a post mortem and died displaying the symptoms of puerperal fever. Semmelweis realised that despite hand washing, medical students were carrying infective body particles from the post mortem. He escalated handwashing to include chlorinated lime, with an immediate 90% reduction in mortality rates. Sadly, his criticism of the medical profession's hygiene and inability to evidence his theories lost him his career (and in time his mental health too). Louis Pasteur later provided the evidence for all that Semmelweis had described and called it antisepsis, providing his own detailed theories around germs and disease.

Hand decontamination

Two categories of bacteria commonly exist on the hands: resident and transient (Muse Health, 2021). Resident bacteria are the harmless microbes that live permanently on the skin. Transient bacteria are those that attach themselves to the hands during daily living.

They can only survive typically between one and three hours, but as there may be as many as 10 million on your fingertips alone they can still spread significantly (Muse Health, 2021). Fortunately, with appropriate hand hygiene numbers of HAIs can be halved (WHO, 2021).

The NHS England (2024) Manual on Infection Prevention and Control advocates five points at which hand hygiene is required. These are listed next with examples of how they should be applied during the physical examination:

1 **Before touching the patient**: on entering the room, before touching the newborn.
2 **Before clean or aseptic procedures**: before physical elements of the examination and if there is a known risk or suspicion of infection.
3 **After body fluid exposure risk**: dribbling, posset, vomit, sneeze, nappy change, blood or any exudate, but also when dressing or undressing, examining the mouth digitally, assessing femoral pulses or developmental dysplasia of the hips and examination of the groin, genitalia or anus.
4 **After touching the patient**: on completion of the physical examination.
5 **After touching the patient's immediate surroundings**: on leaving the room, apply hand gel outside the door before moving on to your next task. In any situation of source isolation nursing or known infection risk, the hands should be fully washed again when leaving the room.

Hand washing and alcohol gel techniques (Figure 29.1)

Typically the hands will be washed with soap and water, but a gel hand rub can be used if the hands are visibly dirty. Gloves and aprons are not routinely required, but this should be decided on an individual basis after assessing any potential infection risk.

Personal hand care

Hands should be examined daily for signs of broken skin, inflammation or torn cuticles (NICE, 2017b). Moisturising prevents drying and cracking from frequent hand washing and alcohol gel use. Nails must be short, smoothly filed and free from nail varnish, extensions or additions. A flat ring band does not prevent good hand hygiene, but clothing below the elbow and all other jewellery (including watches) can both contaminate and interfere with washing and should be removed (NHS England, 2020).

Recognising neonatal infection

Early identification enables appropriate management for the health of the infant and prevention of spread. The history and risk factors will act as indicators and the signs may include:

- Sleepiness with poor feeding.
- Inflammation, redness or an area of localised heat.
- Localised serous fluid or a purulent exudate.
- Vomiting and/or diarrhoea.
- Systemic temperature raised above 38 °C or unstable.
- Increased or reduced respirations or respiratory distress.
- Jitteriness or seizures.
- An area of swelling and/or tenderness.
- Bradycardia.
- Jaundice.
- Apnoea or shock.
- Blood-stained urine (not pseudo-menstruation or urates).

30 Relevant history and risk factors

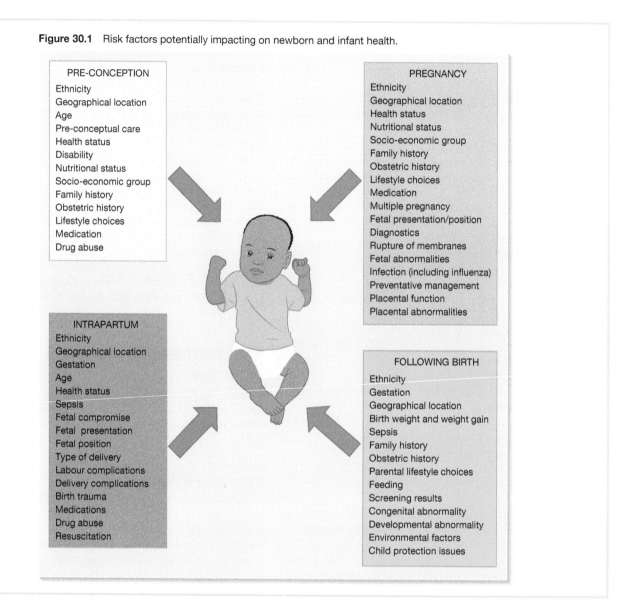

Figure 30.1 Risk factors potentially impacting on newborn and infant health.

PRE-CONCEPTION
Ethnicity
Geographical location
Age
Pre-conceptual care
Health status
Disability
Nutritional status
Socio-economic group
Family history
Obstetric history
Lifestyle choices
Medication
Drug abuse

PREGNANCY
Ethnicity
Geographical location
Health status
Nutritional status
Socio-economic group
Family history
Obstetric history
Lifestyle choices
Medication
Multiple pregnancy
Fetal presentation/position
Diagnostics
Rupture of membranes
Fetal abnormalities
Infection (including influenza)
Preventative management
Placental function
Placental abnormalities

INTRAPARTUM
Ethnicity
Geographical location
Gestation
Age
Health status
Sepsis
Fetal compromise
Fetal presentation
Fetal position
Type of delivery
Labour complications
Delivery complications
Birth trauma
Medications
Drug abuse
Resuscitation

FOLLOWING BIRTH
Ethnicity
Gestation
Geographical location
Birth weight and weight gain
Sepsis
Family history
Obstetric history
Parental lifestyle choices
Feeding
Screening results
Congenital abnormality
Developmental abnormality
Environmental factors
Child protection issues

This chapter aims to help with the identification and analysis of factors within the personal history that may indicate risk. The possible areas of risk are summarised in Figure 30.1 and enlarged on in what follows.

Socio-economic and demographic

Ethnicity: Numerous studies support inequalities in neonatal morbidity and mortality linked to ethnicity, race and colour, including reduced fetal growth, prematurity, low birth weight, chromosomal disorders, birth defects and seizures for Black and minority ethnic groups (Ely and Driscoll, 2019; Lissenkova et al., 2022; Matoba and Collins, 2017).
• **National and international variations**: Differences in access to health support, education and genetics impact on morbidity and

mortality (e.g. higher levels of spina bifida in Wales than in the rest of the United Kingdom).
• **Age**: Teenagers and those of advanced maternal age have increased adverse perinatal health and chromosomal abnormalities in the baby.
• **Disability**: This may be physical/motor (e.g. arthritis, paraplegia, amputation, deformity), sensory (e.g. hearing, sight, speech), intellectual (e.g. learning difficulties, Down syndrome), developmental (e.g. cerebral palsy, autism, spina bifida), mental health (e.g. anxiety, schizophrenia, depression) or visceral (affecting internal organs, e.g. diabetes, epilepsy, asthma). These may impact on parenting abilities, parenting styles and support requirements.
• **BMI/diet**: Raised body mass index (BMI) is linked to neonatal macrosomia, birth trauma and hypoglycaemia. Low BMI impacts attachment and can lead to feeding difficulties.

- **Substance abuse**: Fetal alcohol syndrome or drug withdrawal and neonatal abstinence syndrome.
- **Smoker**: Intrauterine growth retardation (IUGR), hypoxia, prematurity, hypertonia, irritability, increased risk of SIDs.
- **Economic constraints**: Lower- and middle-income families have increased neonatal mortality (Thomson et al., 2021).
- **Consanguinity**: This increases the risk of congenital cardiac anomalies.
- **Domestic abuse and child abuse**: These lead to an increased risk of fetal injury or neonatal neglect, abuse or trauma.
- **Learning difficulties**: These lead to an increased risk of neonatal prematurity and low birth weight, as well as increased parental mental health issues, abuse and socio-economic deprivation plus delayed development of parenting skills.

Family

- **Sibling health**: Reoccurrence of conditions is likely (e.g. cardiac conditions increase 2–3% with one sibling, 50% with two siblings affected).
- **Relatives** (maternal or paternal): Risk increases with any relative, but particularly a first-degree relative, with congenital or developed health concerns. The full history may not be known (e.g. for a single parent, pregnancy supported by donor sperm or a rape victim).
- **Child protection issues**: There is a high risk if the abuser is still within the family.

Screening and diagnostic

- **Rhesus status, blood group and antibody results**: Risk of haemolytic disease of the newborn (HDN), pathological jaundice.
- **HIV status**: Preventative management reduces mother–child transmission to 1–2%, but there is a greater risk of other sexually transmitted infections, hepatitis, tuberculosis, neonatal toxaemia, anaemia and neutropenia.
- **Hepatitis**: Risk of chronic hepatitis if not preventatively managed.
- **Rubella**: Risk of congenital rubella syndrome.
- **Sickle cell**: Risk of tissue hypoxia.
- **Thalassaemia**: Risk of life-threatening anaemia.
- **Ultrasonography**:
  - *Dating scan*: gestation, chromosomal abnormality (absent nasal bone).
  - *Nuchal translucency*: chromosomal abnormality, congenital heart disease.
  - *Ultrasound markers* (echogenic bowel, ventriculomegaly, dilated renal pelves): chromosomal abnormality and/or pathology.
  - *Growth scans*: IUGR.
  - *Polyhydramnios*: duodenal/oesophageal atresia, oligohydramnios, premature rupture of membranes (PROM), growth restriction, infection, renal pathology.
  - *Fetal sex*: X or Y chromosomal sex-linked conditions.
- **Triple and quadruple tests**: Chromosomal abnormalities.
- **Diagnostics** (amniocentesis, CVS, cordocentesis): Chromosomal abnormalities, isoimmunisation, trauma.

Medical, surgical and mental

- **Medical**: Metabolic (diabetes, thyroidism), endocrine (pituitary or adrenal), renal, hypertension, cardiac, venereal, seizures.
- **Medication**: Positive (folic acid), negative effects (thalidomide).
- **Psychological/psychiatric**: Psychotropic medication withdrawal, fetal abnormalities (cardiac, neural tube, cleft palate, floppy baby syndrome), child protection issues.

Antenatal

- **Delayed booking/poor attendance**: Socio-economic risks greater.
- **Fundal height**: Identification of reduced growth.
- **Presentation after 36 weeks' gestation**: Breech presentation (even if vertex at birth), risk of DDH.
- **Anti D**: HDN prevention, following haemorrhage.
- **Multiple pregnancy**: All risks increase.
- **Placental insufficiency** (haemorrhage, reduced movements, pre-eclampsia): Anoxia, meconium.
- **Infection**: Risk of fetal infection (e.g. GBS, syphilis) or abnormality (e.g. rubella, cytomegalovirus, influenza).

Intrapartum and birth

- **Maternal pyrexia and fetal tachycardia**: Risk for neonatal infection.
- **Pre-labour or prolonged rupture of membranes**: Risk of serious neonatal infection is 1% (NICE, 2023b).
- **Meconium liquor**: Risk of meconium aspiration syndrome, respiratory compromise (NICE, 2023b).
- **Presentation/position**: Risk of DDH, trauma, adverse moulding.
- **Birth trauma**: Risk of bruising, jaundice, nerve damage, bone fractures.
- **Precipitate delivery**: Risk of tentorial tears, facial congestion.
- **Gestation**: Risk of prematurity, postmaturity.
- **Fetal compromise** (blood gases, cardiac monitoring): Anoxia.
- **Instrumental/operative delivery**: Risk of birth trauma, jaundice.
- **Medication**: e.g. antibiotic therapy for GBS, magnesium sulphate (hypermagnesaemia) – reduced tone and inactivity, sodium – jaundice.

Early neonatal

- **Apgar**: Resuscitation, transition to extrauterine life.
- **Weight centile**: ≥90th – trauma, hypoglycaemia, ≤10th – IUGR.
- **Head circumference**: Microcephaly, hydrocephaly, abnormal moulding, cephalhaematoma, haemorrhage.
- **Signs of sepsis**: High, low or unstable temperature; respiratory problems; bradycardia; tachycardia; poor tone; poor feeding; unresponsive; seizures; jaundice; vomiting.
- **Screening results** (Kleihauer, Coombs, hearing, blood spot): Isoimmunisation, metabolic disorders, haemoglobinopathies.
- **Feeding**: Poor or incorrect (e.g. hypoglycaemia, jaundice, dehydration, hypernatraemia, vomiting).
- **Bowel movements, urine stream**: Physical abnormalities, renal disease, dehydration (urates), infection, feeding problems.

31 Feeding

Box 31.1 Soft cues for demand feeding.

Rapid eye movement (REM)
Stirring from sleep
Increased movements
Fidgeting
Rooting reflex seen
Sucking reflex seen
Sucking sounds heard
Actual sucking of finger/hand

Box 31.2 Late cues (to be avoided).

Crying

↓

Increasing distress

↓

Newborn releasing cortisol (stress hormone)

Box 31.3 Signs of good latching.

✓ No pain on feeding
✓ Lying chest to chest
✓ Wide open mouth
✓ Lips curled out
✓ Areola fully in mouth (or more visible above than below)
✓ Head tilted back slightly
✓ Cheeks puffed out
✓ Sucking and swallowing
✓ Breasts emptying
✓ Weight gaining

Box 31.4 Decontamination of formula feeding equipment.

There are three main methods used for decontamination of formula feeding equipment:
• Boiling
• Chemical treatment
• Steam (electrical or microwave)

Figure 31.1 Good latching.
Source: Wren Meinberg/UnSplash.

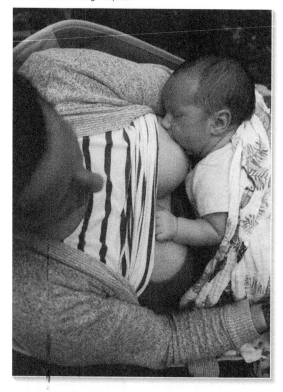

Box 31.5 Essentials of formula feed preparation.

1 Clean/decontaminate all equipment
2 Wash hands and work surfaces
3 Make feeds one at a time as needed
4 Boil fresh tap water and leave to cool to 70 °C (up to 30 minutes)
5 Pour water into bottle to correct level
6 Fill scoop provided with loose powder – do not compress; level off using knife
7 Secure teat without contaminating it
8 Add cap and shake to dissolve powder
9 Cool before feeding

Physical Examination of the Newborn at a Glance, Second Edition. Dr Lyn Dolby and Denise (Dee) Campbell.
© 2025 John Wiley & Sons Ltd. Published 2025 by John Wiley & Sons Ltd.

The feeding decision will already have been made by the time of the physical examination. It is important that the examiner is not judgemental and respects individual choice, with awareness that formula feeding may occur because of a contraindication to breastfeeding. This chapter concentrates on the assessment that feeding has been initiated/established and is progressing well, as well as recognition of the most common feeding problems.

Contraindications to breastfeeding

Sensitivity is required around situations in which breastfeeding may be the first choice but where breastfeeding (or milk production) is not possible, is delayed or is contraindicated. Additional support may be needed to express breastmilk and establish a milk supply if breastfeeding is only delayed.

Maternal
- HIV infection.
- Antiretroviral medication.
- Human T-cell lymphotropic virus types 1 and 2.
- Drug or substance abuse.
- Chemotherapy.
- Radiotherapy (treatment or diagnostic therapy).
- Active tuberculosis.
- Breast tissue damage, e.g. following trauma or breast augmentation.
- Bilateral mastectomy.
- Breast abscess.
- Active herpes simplex lesions on the breast.
- Active varicella zoster lesions on the breast.
- Coma.

Newborn
- Physical abnormality affecting the ability to feed (e.g. oesophageal atresia).
- Metabolic abnormality affecting tolerance to milk (e.g. galactosemia).
- Acute illness or infection affecting the ability to feed.
- Prematurity.

Initiation and establishment of feeding

Positive signs: general
- Feeding commenced as soon after birth as possible.
- Demand feeding is practised associated with early feeding cues (Boxes 31.1 and 31.2).
- Newborn is waking naturally for feeds.
- Newborn is settling between feeds – cluster feeding is possible (a number of feeds in quick succession before a longer gap).
- No vomiting – dribbles and possets are possible.
- Normal micturition and stools – frequency, colour and consistency.
- Contented mother and newborn with evidence of bonding.
- Initial weight loss is no greater than 10% of birth weight and regaining from 4 days – back to or above birthweight by 14 days.
- No signs of newborn dehydration.

Breastfeeding specific
- Both breasts at each feed for unrestricted time period.
- 8–12 feeds per day.

- Progress from colostrum to milk by 24–72 hours.
- Filling of breasts between/before a feed (from 48 to 72 hours).
- Newborn latching well (Box 31.3 and Figure 31.1).
- Breasts emptying during feeds (4 days onwards).
- No supplementary feeding required.
- Nipples and breasts unproblematic.

Formula feeding specific
- 6–10 feeds per day and settling between feeds.
- Sucking and pausing are intermittent during feeds.
- Small feeds initially build to 150–200 mL/kg/day by 1 week old.
- Air flow back into bottle during paused feeding.
- Correct approaches to decontamination of equipment and making of feeds (Boxes 31.4 and 31.5).

Common problems

A full history should be taken around feeding, including patterns, length, frequency, positioning of infant, air swallowing and winding. Examine for signs of infection, obstruction or ill health, including frequency, colour, smell and amounts of urine and stool passed. If breastfeeding, examine the breasts for signs of infection or sore nipples. If formula feeding, assess decontamination of equipment, preparation and temperature of feed – by all individuals involved.

Excessive weight gain
This is weight gain above the expectation of a centile chart or where a significant jump is seen. Distinguish between correct demand feeding and incorrectly feeding whenever a newborn is fretful (as opposed to hungry). Over-concentrated formula, supplements, early weaning and over-feeding (pushing additional or longer feeds on an already satisfied newborn) can result in excessive weight gain.

Failure to thrive
This is inadequate weight gain after allowing for initial weight loss and variable weight gain patterns. A fall in weight gain is of greater concern than regular weight gain along a low centile. It may be caused by incorrect feeding (over-diluted feeds, poor latching), inadequate feeding (drowsy infant, abuse or poor parenting), poor absorption (allergy or abnormality) or excessive elimination (diarrhoea or vomiting).

Vomiting
Small regurgitations or dribbles linked to feeding or winding are normal (possets). Errors in reconstitution of formula feeds, air swallowing, over-stimulation, over-feeding, infection, allergy, food intolerance, reflux, hernia or obstruction can lead to vomiting. It is important to assess the frequency, amount, colour and pattern of occurrence alongside the general health of the newborn.

Constipation
This is passage of a hard, dry stool. Infants may go 2–3 days without passing a stool and still not be constipated. Constipation causes include dehydration, over-concentrated formula milk, incorrect feeding, stenosis (bowel or anus) or disease (e.g. Hirschsprung's disease).

32 Excretion

Figure 32.1 Meconium.
Source: Jeremy Kemp/Wikimedia Commons/Public domain.

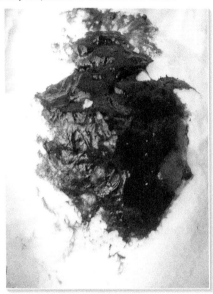

Figure 32.2 Changing stool.
Source: Bart Van Gheluwe/Wikimedia Commons/CC BY SA 3.0.

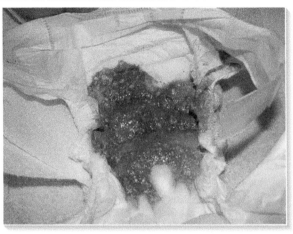

Figure 32.4 Formula-fed stool – semi-formed.

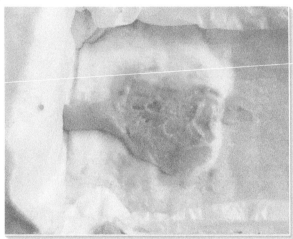

Figure 32.3 Breastfed stool.

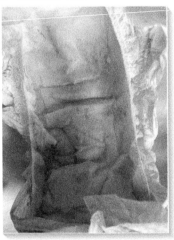

Figure 32.5 Hydronephrosis (level 1 left; level 4 right).

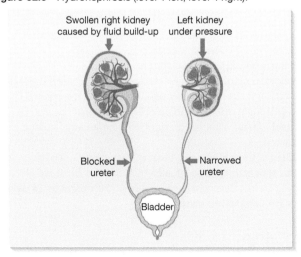

Box 32.1 Symptoms of urinary tract infection – some or all may be present.

- Hot to touch/pyrexia
- Not eating as well as normal
- Vomiting
- Irritability/pain on handling
- Cloudy, blood-stained, darker urine
- More sleepy than normal
- Diarrhoea (difficult to determine if breastfed – note changes from normal)
- More offensive stool

Physical Examination of the Newborn at a Glance, Second Edition. Dr Lyn Dolby and Denise (Dee) Campbell.
© 2025 John Wiley & Sons Ltd. Published 2025 by John Wiley & Sons Ltd.

This chapter details normal excretion and includes information about the more common problems that may occur, their symptoms and their causes. The focus is on excretion from the bladder and bowel (abnormal excretion from the mouth, nose and lungs is included in their specific chapters). The relevant history and risk factors should be considered before examination: family history, anomaly screening, oligohydramnios and meconium liquor. The examination benefits from knowledge of normal genitalia, patency of the external anal meatus, kidney palpation and details of the feeding pattern. It is essential that the number and nature of bladder and bowel movements are ascertained, as well as any vomiting or abdominal distension preceding the examination.

Bowel

In utero, from 16 weeks' gestation, meconium has formed in the colon. A mixture of epithelial, amniotic and blood cells within the digestive tract, along with mucus, bile, amniotic fluid and fatty acids, has been acted on by digestive enzymes, resulting in this greeny-black substance (Figure 32.1). The presence of meconium helps to keep the colon patent along its length as the fetus grows. Unlike the bladder, the bowel is not typically active in utero. Meconium may be passed by the postmature fetus or during episodes of fetal compromise. Reduced oxygen levels cause muscle relaxation, including the anal sphincter, and meconium escapes into the liquor.

The consistency of any meconium in the liquor changes over time, becoming more diluted; this is affected by the amount of meconium passed and the time. Degrees and consistency of meconium are classified as significant (if dark green-black and thick and tenacious, or containing lumps) or insignificant, with management in utero, at birth and postnatally determined accordingly (NICE, 2023b).

Typically, meconium is first passed in the 24 hours following birth and clears from the system in approximately 48 hours. By day 2–3 a green-brown, changing stool becomes evident (Figure 32.2). This is when the lighter-coloured stool of the feeding baby appears seedy and stained from the traces of meconium. After this the stool is affected by the type of feeding:
- **Breastfeeding** (Figure 32.3): loose, bright yellow-green, inoffensive and often with a mustard seed appearance. Huge range in frequency is normal, from 1 stool every 3 days to 10 per day.
- **Formula feeding** (Figure 32.4): pale, semi-formed, with a sour smell. Frequency is 4–6 per day, with increased risk of firm or constipated stool.

Common abnormalities
- **Constipation**: difficulties passing firm stool. Infrequent passage of stool is rarely constipation unless accompanied by severe straining, anal twitching and signs of discomfort. Increase fluids by breastfeeding more frequently; check formula feed mix.
- **Delayed passage of stool**: consider meconium plug, meconium ileus, Hirschsprung's disease, cystic fibrosis and imperforate anus.
- **Diarrhoea**: increased frequency and runniness of stool. May be a result of infection, maternal diet, fore–hind milk imbalance, food allergy.
- **Haematochezia**: fresh blood in stool. May be linked to food allergies from mother (lactose intolerance), infection or fissures caused by constipation.
- **Melaena**: partially digested blood from upper digestive tract in stool; stool appears black (after meconium stage).
- **Mucus**: can be normal in a breastfeeding baby. If it persists, ensure fore and hind milk are taken in balance and consider food allergy to something the mother is eating.
- **Pus**: white cells in a microbiology tested stool; result of inflammation or infection.
- **White stool**: may be caused by a medication taken. Also consider anaemia, lack of bile, cyst or tumour, lactose intolerance or galactosemia.

Kidneys and bladder

Bladder filling and emptying begin in utero for the normal healthy newborn, but the placenta remains the organ of excretion. The kidneys remain immature at birth, rapidly maturing over the first week. Poor glomerular filtration initially causes difficulties in concentrating the urine (with reabsorption of sodium and imbalanced fluid loss) and may result in urine having a cloudy appearance at birth. Micturition for the newborn is a basic reflex controlled by the spinal cord in response to stretching of the trigone within the bladder. The trigone is a sensitive triangle in the wall of the bladder between the two ureters and the urethra. At birth, the bladder can only hold around 15 mL of urine and urine output is about 0.5 mL/kg per hour, rising to 2–3 mL/kg from day 2 (Sinha et al., 2018).

The first urine passed is normally within 24 hours and would typically be pale, straw coloured and inoffensive. A reddish-brown, powdery discharge (urates) sometimes occurs as a result of mild dehydration, slight acidosis (uric acid) and fluid imbalance. This is insignificant unless it continues beyond the first few days. Occasionally there may even be no urine passed in the first 48 hours, but if the infant is alert, feeding well and there is no vomiting or abdominal swelling, this is unlikely to be a problem. It may just be that urine has been missed within the stool of a dirty nappy, but a square of kitchen roll or tissue placed in the nappy will help monitor urine output.

Common abnormalities
- **Hydronephrosis** (Figure 32.5): fluid filling the kidney. This is due to blockage or restricted flow of urine away from the kidney, most commonly a narrowed ureter. May resolve spontaneously after birth, but severe cases require surgery. Incidence is around 1 in 600 births.
- **Haematuria**: blood in urine. Visible blood should not be present. Investigation is needed for signs of renal failure, infection (Box 32.1), tumour, trauma or coagulation disorders.
- **Oliguria**: failure to make/pass urine. May be due to developmental complication, obstruction, neurological damage, renal agenesis or cardiopulmonary disease.
- **Urine dribbling/leakage**: due to posterior urethral valves (male infants only with a 1 in 5000–8000 incidence). Partial blockage of the urethra leads to an enlarged bladder under pressure and dribbling urine slowly. Untreated, back flow damage will cause renal failure.
- **Urinary tract infection** (Box 32.1): more common in boys than girls. Typically blood borne and more likely with abnormalities, but may also be caused by ascending infection.

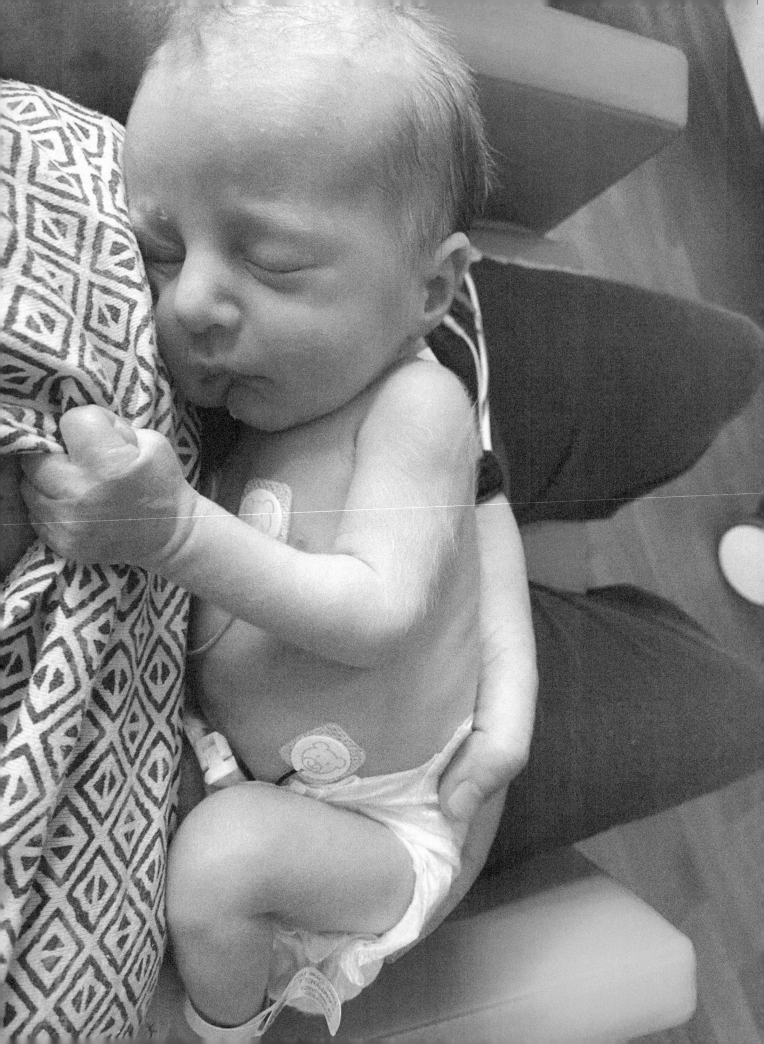

Top-to-toe physical examination

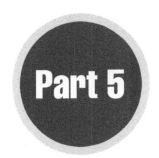

Part 5

Chapters

33 Newborn and infant physical examination: overview

Table 33.1 Key aspects of the newborn and physical examination.

Aspect	Observe and assess the following elements	
Predisposing factors	Investigate *Recorded history*: family, antenatal, intrapartum and maternal/neonatal progress or concerns since birth *Ask parent(s)*: for information on any concerns or family history relevant to their baby that they wish to discuss	
Colour	Well perfused	Jaundiced? TcB or SBR performed? Results?
Head	Skull and fontanelles Facial features and ears/signs of dysmorphia Hearing screening performed?	Head circumference Appropriate use of tape measure (cm towards brow) to aid in consistency of measurement
Neck/clavicles	Tumours, webbing, fractures	
Palate	Digital and visual inspection	Teeth, tongue and/or lip tie
Posture/behaviour	Flexion, tone, response to touch and handling Alertness and general demeanour	
Cardiac	Use an infant-sized stethoscope and auscultate with both diaphragm and bell Apex rate: capillary refill, heaves and thrills	Brachial and femoral pulses Pedal pulses (if required) Cord bloods taken? Results?
Respiratory	Note rate, clear air entry?	Recession, grunting, nasal flaring
Chest	Shape Nipple number and position	Neonatal gynaecomastia
Abdomen	Masses, tone	Kidneys palpated
Umbilicus	Clamp secure, on	Inflammation/discharge Hernia
Upper limbs	No. of digits counted L and R Palm creases	Bone integrity Movement, interdigital webbing
Lower limbs	Bone integrity No. of digits counted L and R Plantar creases	Movement Talipes Interdigital webbing
Genitalia	*Male* Epstein pearls, epispadias Smooth urine flow Penis length/chordee Hydrocoele, testes ↓↓	*Female* Appearance Pseudo-menstruation Mucous Tags
Hips	Allis sign Leg length (do not press down on knees, there is a natural stricture behind the knee that should not be forcibly stretched)	Ortolani and Barlow's manoeuvres L and R = 'stable'? Single hip anomaly – note if 'unstable' or 'dislocated' etc.
Spine	Integrity (link with how baby moves arms and legs)	Sacral dimple/hair tufts Naevus/abnormal skin patches
Eyes	Appearance Discharge: sticky or purulent Alert, fixation	Red reflex normal: L and R noted as normal Use of ophthalmoscope Subconjunctival haemorrhage or trauma from delivery
Skin	Condition Rashes	Birth marks Trauma
Anus	Appearance, position Patency	Meconium passed and date Changing stool or unusual consistency (e.g. pale, green) – link with abdominal findings
Urine	Urine passed and date noted (link with abdominal findings)	Urates passed
Reflexes	Suckling, gag and blink Moro (noted if bilateral and equal) Incurving (Galant reflex)	Stepping/placing Grasp Babinski/plantar flexion
Vaccination	Anti-D; BCG required or given?	
Feeding	Method, frequency and progress	If formula milk – which one? Quantity?
Health promotion information	Immunisations – when these commence and where information can be accessed Parental health activities – car seats, pram systems, smoking, safer sleeping and 'tummy time' Signs of ill health and where to seek advice Next screening examination with the GP – infant examination at 6 to 8 weeks	

Physical Examination of the Newborn at a Glance, Second Edition. Dr Lyn Dolby and Denise (Dee) Campbell.
© 2025 John Wiley & Sons Ltd. Published 2025 by John Wiley & Sons Ltd.

At times an abnormality not detected during pregnancy or soon after birth will present during the neonatal period, even in an apparently healthy baby due to the developmental changes occurring within the neonate. Occasionally one of the parents voices a concern about a particular issue, or during the examination the practitioner finds an anomaly. At these moments the level of professional sensitivity, knowledge and understanding employed will make a significant difference to the parent(s) as the initial impact of the issue of concern sinks in. However, it is paramount that if anomalies are found these concerns must be expressed to the parent(s), followed by an explanation regarding the action that will be taken. It should never be the case that a particular anomaly or specific signs and symptoms are noted and the baby referred to the paediatric team without first discussing the reason for doing so with the parent(s) – this would be wholly unacceptable practice.

The assessment of neonatal health and well-being commences with the initial examination at birth and continues with the daily examination of the baby. A systematic examination of the newborn (PHE, 2021a) is offered for all babies within 72 hours of birth. A second systematic examination is offered again when the baby is 6 to 8 weeks of age with the GP. At times the newborn examination may not have occurred within 72 hours of birth, particularly if the baby is ill. This must be clearly documented and all staff (including the parent(s) when appropriate) must be informed that the examination has not yet been performed. It is the responsibility of the practitioners to offer the newborn examination when appropriate and for community staff to check that the examination has been performed. Also, parents need to be informed during the newborn examination who they should contact if they have an urgent concern, as opposed to who they should seek information from for a more minor issue.

Each NHS Trust site will have its own specific criteria in place regarding who can complete the examination, depending on the baby's condition, age or already identified concerns. For example, midwives who have received training to enable them to conduct the examination of the newborn (either post registration or as part of the initial pre-registration midwifery programme of study) can usually only do so if the baby is ≥37 weeks' gestation and/or has reached a particular growth centile by birth. The local protocols and guidelines for the practice area must be taken into account and it is the practitioner's responsibility to be fully conversant with these.

Before the examination

The practitioner should investigate the notes for predisposing factors, maternal blood results, scans and identification of conditions that have been noted (management protocols may already be in place). At times this information will mean that the baby must be examined by a member of the paediatric team and the parent(s) need to be made aware of the rationale for this.

As with all examinations, the parent(s) should always be informed about what the examination process entails and their understanding of this assessed whether they speak and understand English or not. This is not only so that the parent(s) can make an informed decision in relation to consent, but they also need to understand the examination findings and the information that is shared with them throughout the examination. Therefore, the use of an interpreting or translation service may be necessary in some circumstances.

The examination should be performed where it can be easily witnessed by the parent(s), so not on a resuscitaire where the parent(s) may need to stand to see what is happening, which for those who have had a caesarean section can prove difficult. Natural daylight is preferably (easier to detect cyanosis, some birth marks and level of jaundice). Hands should be washed and dried prior to the examination and everything required should be close by (e.g. nappy and baby clothes). The examination should be performed quickly and comprehensively, only uncovering the part of the baby being examined and re-covering the baby as soon as is practicable in order that they do not become unduly cold and fretful. The examiner should be professional and gentle in their actions and mindful that part of their task is to provide a good role model, for example a baby's arms and legs are not 'handles' to be used for turning the baby over. The stethoscope or ophthalmoscope should not be placed in the cot with the baby or the nappy when removed placed near the baby's head, as both are aspects of poor infection control.

It is necessary to remember that parents observe the examiner's actions, facial expressions and the words used and how they are spoken. Therefore, if the baby is fidgety and it is taking a while to perform auscultation of the heart, reassure the parent(s). Likewise, if an anomaly is found, the parent(s) should be informed at the time, particularly if urgent action is required. When a referral is required but no urgent action is needed, the finding should be discussed again with the parent(s) so that they have a clear idea what will happen next.

Examination of the newborn: process

The examination of the newborn should include the aspects and elements identified in Table 33.1, following a systematic process in order not to miss any part of the examination. Always commence the examination by asking the parent(s) for their impression of their baby's health and if they have any concerns, as these may include issues that have arisen during the antenatal period. Parent(s) should also be asked if they have any family history of heart, kidney or hip conditions **from birth**, as occasionally something that has become 'normal' for the parent(s) is not highlighted at booking.

It is always best to commence the examination with auscultation of the heart if possible, even if the baby is in a parent's arms, after which continue with the top-to-toe examination. The hands should be in gentle contact with the baby most of the time, allowing the baby to gradually wake and preventing over-stimulation. Certain aspects of the examination such as auscultation of the heart, eye examination and hip assessment can prove impossible with a crying baby. Sometimes the examination should be temporarily abandoned if the baby is too distressed until the reason for the distress is resolved (e.g. pain, needs feeding, has been over-stimulated).

Examining the eyes sometimes proves difficult at this stage of life as the baby, unless fully alert, is more likely to keep their eyes closed or only partly open. Use of the doll's eye reflex, placing the baby over a parent's shoulder or on their knee, or even walking into a darker area of the room and closing the curtains can help. A baby who is gently spoken to will tend to be calmer and more alert as they concentrate on the source of vocalisation. If patience is employed there should be no need to 'force' the eyelids open, which can cause minor trauma.

The hip assessment usually occurs just before the baby is gently picked up and turned over in order to view the back and elicit the walk reflex. On turning the baby over, perform the reflexes first, as some babies become accustomed to lying over the hand when their back and spine is examined and are then reluctant to demonstrate the reflexes. If the baby is placed back in the cot after the examination, follow safer sleeping guidance.

After the examination

Immediately after the examination the findings and salient aspects must be discussed while the parent(s)' attention is directed towards their baby. They should be fully informed of the findings of the examination and if issues of concern have arisen what will happen next or why immediate action was required. All aspects of health promotion should be discussed (see Table 33.1). All findings and discussions should be documented in full within the neonatal record, the Trust digital system, the SMaRT4NIPE (S4N) system and the PCHR.

34 Neurological assessment: overview

Table 34.1 Normal stages of rising consciousness.

Sleep state	Sleep	Baby's movements/activity
State 1	Deep sleep	Regular breathing, eyes closed with no eye movement visible, no spontaneous activity but may make regular jerky movements. External stimuli produce slightly delayed startle motion that is rapidly suppressed
State 2	Light sleep (active sleep)	Eyes are closed, but rapid eye movements are visible with the eyes opening for a brief moment. Baby makes random movements and often responds to internal and external stimuli, which frequently provoke a change in sleep state. Respiration can be irregular and suckling movements occur intermittently
State 3	Drowsy (semi-dozing)	Eyes may be open, but any response to external stimuli is delayed. However, sleep state may change after stimuli. Slight startles may occur, but movement is smooth
State 4	Quiet awake	Baby is alert, focused and attentive. Other stimuli may distract the focus of attention but the response is delayed. Motor activity is minimal. Learning activity is high
State 5	Fussing	Eyes are open with considerable bodily activity. Reacts to external stimuli with increased activity. Fussy vocalisation may be heard, may quieten to sound of parent's voice or cuddling
State 6	Crying	Intense crying with lots of activity. May take time to quieten with cuddling or consoling activities

Table 34.2 Congenital malformations of the neurological system.

Anencephaly	The baby is born without part of the brain and skull
Cranial encephalocele	Rare condition where the brain and membranes protrude through an opening in the skull in a sac-like bulge
Hydrocephaly	Build-up of fluid within the brain that elevates intracranial pressure, putting pressure on the brain tissue that can cause damage. Hydrocephalus can be fatal
Microcephaly	Abnormal smallness of the head associated with incomplete brain development
Megalencephaly	Unusually enlarged brain (unilateral or bilateral) often resulting in neurological and developmental problems
Agenesis of corpus callosum	Rare, congenital brain defect where the corpus callosum (a band of tissue that connects the left and right sides of the brain) does not develop normally. Severity of symptoms vary from very mild to life changing
Spina bifida (occulta)	Mildest form caused by incomplete closure of the neural tube, which causes a hole in some of the vertebrae. Can result in spinal cord and nerve damage, which may cause mild to severe disabilities
Meningocele	Spinal vertebrae do not close completely, allowing a protrusion of the meninges through the hole that has been created
Dandy-Walker syndrome	Congenital condition where the cerebellum does not develop normally

Box 34.1 Key neurological alarm signals.

- Persistent irritability
- **Seizures** – most start 12–48 hours after birth, with 50% caused by hypoxic–ischaemic encephalopathy, or to a lesser extent focal cerebral infarction or viral or bacterial infection
- Difficulty in feeding
- Persistent deviation of head or eyes
- Asymmetry in posture and movements that is persistent
- **Opisthotonus** – severe hyperextension and spasticity in which an individual's head, neck and spinal column enter into a complete 'bridging' or 'arching' position
- Floppiness or, conversely, hyperexcitability, over-active reflexes or seizures
- Abnormal cry
- Apathy
- Convulsions
- Persistent setting-sun sign, often associated with elevated intracranial pressure (e.g. as in hydrocephaly)
- Respiratory difficulties, apnoea, changes or loss of variability in heart rate

Assessing the neurological status and behavioural responses of a baby from birth may give an indication of potential problems relating to future developmental and/or cognitive ability. Most babies born prematurely or who have significant health issues at birth will be assessed by the senior paediatric team and their care managed according to the findings. Babies born with dysmorphic features, excessive moulding or unusual appearance of the suture lines, naevus flammeus (port wine stain), hypo- or hypertonia, odd eye movements or unusual behaviours will need immediate referral to a senior paediatrician. For the term, apparently healthy

Physical Examination of the Newborn at a Glance, Second Edition. Dr Lyn Dolby and Denise (Dee) Campbell.
© 2025 John Wiley & Sons Ltd. Published 2025 by John Wiley & Sons Ltd.

baby, there is a need to assess if the baby's responses are appropriate for the gestational age and condition (Brazelton and Nugent, 2011) and there is usually no necessity to assess gestational age as one might do with a premature or very small baby. What is important are good observational skills when observing for the presence of normal neurological responses in a baby. Asking the parent(s)' opinion about their baby's behaviour and response to handling and other stimuli such as sound and light, as well as the sleeping pattern, can provide valuable information for the practitioner.

Sleep patterns

Although a preterm baby may spend much of their time asleep, the cycles between activity and rest, regular and irregular breathing and whether eye movements are visible are not so pronounced as in a term baby. This reflects the latter's maturity, not just physically but also neurologically. The normal term baby will usually move between behavioural states, spending most of their time in quiet and active sleep. Approximately 50 minutes per hour will consist of sleep time, of which 50% will be spent in quiet sleep. Brazelton and Nugent (2011) define the normal sleep pattern as passing through a number of stages or 'states' (Table 34.1) unless this pattern is interrupted, such as when the baby is disturbed.

Body position and activity

The normal body posture for a term baby, whether prone or supine, is well flexed with the head usually lying in the midline and limbs often held in a roughly symmetrical position. Babies with intact neurology typically alternately move their arms and legs. As both palmar and plantar grasp are present in the fetus from 26 weeks' gestation (persisting until approximately 4 months of age), by term the hands are usually tightly closed and often held near the chin or upper part of the body.

Many babies may appear to 'jitter' or startle in their sleep (Table 34.1), but one can easily test if this is normal movement (known as a myoclonic jerk) as opposed to a seizure by holding the limb in question – if it is a normal movement the jitter will stop. With a seizure this will not happen and it may be accompanied by ocular deviation or autonomic changes, such as mottling, or changes in colour or respiratory rate.

When the baby's limbs are moved, there should be obvious muscle resistance and tone. If the baby is pulled to a sitting position, the head may initially lag slightly but the baby should be able to demonstrate movement towards the upright position. Although the baby may not be able to hold their head up for long, the ability to do so will have been demonstrated. Similarly, when lying in ventral suspension over the examiner's hand, the baby should be capable of holding head and legs in alignment with the back. Again, this may only be for a short time and a sleepy baby may not demonstrate this ability. The baby should also be capable of flexing their limbs against gravity. They will also demonstrate neurological reflexes that are appropriate to their gestational age and these are highlighted in Chapter 35.

Crying

Crying is a baby's method of communicating with the world as they try to convey discomfort, hunger or pain. A normal healthy term baby will have a lusty cry that eventually terminates when an appropriate method of solace is given, such as being cuddled close to the chest or over the parent's shoulder. However, it is abnormal for a baby to have a persistent high-pitched or weak cry and this may demonstrate that there is a neurological impact, caused, for example, by drug withdrawal or hypoxic–ischaemic encephalopathy.

Feeding and suckling

The rooting reflex is present by 28 weeks' gestation and suckling begins during week 11. The ability to coordinate suckling and swallowing occurs at approximately 28 weeks' gestation, with strength and coordination of breathing at around 32–34 weeks' gestation. Therefore, if the baby does not appear capable of normal feeding responses, the integrity of the cranial nerves should be tested. The examiner can try to elicit the rooting reflex by gently stroking the upper lip or corner of the mouth. The fifth cranial nerve is involved here as this conducts sensation; nerves 5, 7 and 12 relate to the motor pathways, and swallowing involves nerves 9 and 10. If suckling is absent, the gag reflex can be provoked by gently stroking the soft palate with a finger, which should elicit the appropriate response. However, it should be noted that some neurologically sound babies may have a headache caused by birth trauma and may also be reluctant to feed.

Eyes

A pupillary reflex (pupil reacts to light) can be apparent in the fetus after 30 weeks' and definitely by 35 weeks' gestation. Even a baby of 26 weeks' gestation will respond to light by blinking and can briefly track objects by 34 weeks. Therefore, how the eyes of a term baby react to light, how they move and fixate, can provide important neurological markers. Thus, the pupils of the eyes will usually lie mid position and will generally move together in the same direction. Horizontal divergence is normal until about 6 weeks of age, when the activity of looking and focusing on objects should have provided enough stimuli to strengthen the muscles of the eye and nerve pathways. However, abnormal reactions include constant deviation and persistent strabismus or nystagmus. It is important to note here that vertical deviation is always abnormal, often the result of germinal matrix haemorrhage or intraventricular haemorrhage. Although both of these types of haemorrhage are more likely to occur in preterm babies, it is not unknown for them to occur in the term neonate.

Neurological alarm signals

Congenital malformations of the neurological system are summarised in Table 34.2. Box 34.1 presents a list of the most common signs that all is not well in relation to neurological function. See Fanning (2024) for more detailed information on neurological assessment.

The main causes of neurological compromise requiring referral and/or investigation include the following.

- **Meningitis**: current incidence is 0.21 per 1000 births.
- **Drug withdrawal**: symptoms can occur up to 3 weeks after birth, effects can persist for several months, and withdrawal from methadone is worse than from heroin.
- **Intracranial haemorrhage**: seizures are usually noted and sometimes pyrexia.
- **Hypoxic–ischaemic brain injury**: usually caused by a hypoxic episode during the intrapartum period.
- **Acidosis**: from respiratory failure or metabolic in origin.
- **Hypoglycaemia**: more likely in babies who are small for their gestational age and the effect is heightened with hypoxia.
- **Hypocalcaemia and hyponatraemia**.
- **Hereditary and degenerative central nervous system disease**.
- **Inborn errors of metabolism**: PKU and Galactosaemia.
- **Congenital brain tumours**: most common is astrocytoma.
- **Cerebrovascular malformations**: such as Sturge-Weber syndrome.

35 Reflexes

Table 35.1 Reflexes usually assessed during the examination of the newborn.

Established by	Primitive reflex	Disappears by approximately	Importance
28/32 weeks	Palmer flexion (grasp)	4 months	Maintain contact with parent
28/34 weeks	Rooting	3–4 months	Both assist with searching for and locating food
28/40 weeks	Suck	4–6 months	
32 weeks	Plantar flexion	8–12 months	Initiates foot responses to contact with surfaces
32 weeks	Moro/startle	2–4 months	Initial fight or flight response
34 weeks	Babinski	9–12 months	Similar to plantar flexion
35/40 weeks	Gag	Permanent	Protection of the airways
Birth	Swallow	Permanent	
Birth	Tonic neck reflex	5–7 months	Aid in later hand–eye coordination
35–37 weeks	Step	3 months but returns at approximately 9 months	Initiates leg and foot responses for later crawling and walking
35–37 weeks	Placing	Permanent	
Birth	Incurving or Galant	3–6 months	
Birth	Ventral suspension	–	
Birth	Blinking	Permanent	Protection of the eye

Box 35.1 Activities that assist in natural progression from involuntary to voluntary reflexes.

- Adequate time should be spent flat on the tummy and the back
- Babies and infants should spend minimal amounts of time in car seats, high chairs, pushchairs, bouncers etc., as these encourage the spine into a C-shape rather than the straighter position required for balance and walking
- Babies should be allowed to pass through each developmental stage without being rushed

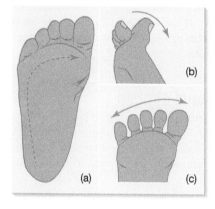

Figure 35.1 (a–c) Babinski's reflex.

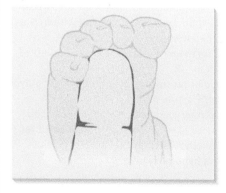

Figure 35.2 Plantar flexion.

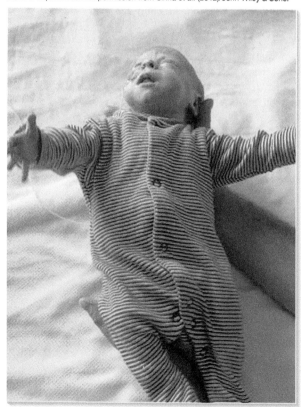

Figure 35.3 Eliciting the Moro reflex.
Source: Reproduced with permission from Sinha et al. (2012)/John Wiley & Sons.

Many of the primary reflexes that can be assessed at birth were initiated during intrauterine life and are often referred to as primitive, locomotor and postural reflexes (Table 35.1). These primitive reflexes are **involuntary** (not voluntary, i.e. 'learned') and are essential for neonatal survival, for example rooting, suckling, swallowing, urinating, grasp and the Moro reflex. **Locomotor** reflexes link to the development of later voluntary movement, for example the step reflex will develop later into 'walking'. Many of the **postural** reflexes develop after approximately 3 months of age and are therefore termed secondary reflexes, but the tonic neck reflex is observable at birth (Modrell and Tadi, 2023). Absence or abnormal reflexes can be a sign of central nervous system (CNS) dysfunction and therefore they are an important part of the initial examination and the NIPE. However, it is important that later as the child develops voluntary reflexes take over, otherwise normal behaviour and activity can be disrupted. Activities that encourage voluntary reflexes can be seen in Box 35.1.

Assessment

During the examination of the newborn, the reflexes in the following sections tend to be observed or elicited as the examination progresses. However, particular reflexes (e.g. Moro and rooting reflexes) may occur spontaneously and a mental note that they have been observed should be made at the time they are observed. It is also easier to elicit or observe responses if the baby is calm and not agitated. Parents are usually very interested in learning what their baby is capable of and the process of their child's development.

Rooting, suck, gag and swallow

If the cheek or corner of the mouth is stroked or touched, the baby will start to open their mouth and turn towards the stimulus. Touching or stroking the lips will encourage the baby to open their mouth wider, allowing a finger or nipple to enter and further encouraging suckling and assessment of strength and coordination. Swallowing movements can be seen and the gag reflex may be elicited when exploring for integrity of the soft palate, as stroking the soft palate will often elicit the gag response.

Head lag

Head lag is not usually routinely performed on a term baby, unless there are other abnormal neurological signs. The baby's arms or hands are held securely while they are raised to a sitting position. The head will momentarily support itself in the midline and will then lag to one side or fall backwards. Eventually, full head control will be achieved as the neck muscles strengthen.

Ventral suspension and incurving (Galant)

A demonstration of ventral suspension can be elicited when the term baby is placed tummy downwards over the hand, and arms and legs will flex in conjunction with the head lifting and rotating. Incurving or the Galant reflex will be observed if a finger is gently drawn down one side of the back, causing the baby's pelvis to curve to the side being tested.

Blinking

Blinking, as in adults, serves to protect the eye from trauma by distributing moisture around the eye and softening the impact of direct contact with objects. Any neurological impact that prevents the eye from closing such as facial nerve palsy will require administration of lubrication (artificial tears) to prevent corneal damage.

Tonic neck reflex ('fencing position')

When the infant is in a supine, neutral position, turn their head to one side. The arm on the side the head is turned to will extend (often with the hand opening), while flexion occurs in the opposite arm and leg. The reflex disappears at approximately 2–4 months of age. An inability or exaggerated response can indicate an abnormality.

Palmer flexion (grasp), Babinski's reflex and plantar flexion

Stroking the palm of the baby's hand with a finger should stimulate palmer flexion, which becomes stronger when an attempt is made to withdraw the finger. The strength of the palmer grasp can be assessed by the examiner pulling their finger towards themselves and observing that the baby's body can lift off the bed.

Babinski's reflex will usually occur straight after plantar flexion has been elicited. The former response is encouraged by drawing the examiner's finger towards the little toe and across the ball of the foot (Figure 35.1a). The toes will extend and flex towards the dorsum of the foot (Figure 35.2b) while splaying apart (Figure 35.1c). If the reflex is consistently absent, it may point to an underlying neurological abnormality. The plantar reflex is easily elicited by applying finger pressure to the ball of the foot just under the toe line, causing a flexion of the toes towards the plantar surface (Figure 35.2). Plantar flexion assists with crawling but disappears to allow the development of stable walking, which cannot easily occur if the toes are flexed.

Moro or startle

The baby should be calm and supported in a supine, neutral position with their hands close to their body (Figure 35.3). The examiner tilts the baby's head forwards towards its chest and then suddenly allows the head to drop backwards a couple of centimetres. Initially the baby's response will be to quickly extend and abduct their arms and the hands will open with the fingers splaying apart. This action will be followed by a slight adduction with accompanying flexion and closing of the hands. Complete absence of this reflex is abnormal and asymmetrical movements may suggest brachial plexus palsy or a bone injury. However, it is possible for the Moro reflex to be elicited even in the event of clavicular fracture where the bone ends are in good apposition to one another, causing little discomfort to the baby.

Stepping and placing

Observing one or other of these reflexes is usually regarded as a positive response. Stepping is best elicited immediately after turning the baby from the supine position to the 'standing' position with the baby's body slightly leaning forwards. Contact between the baby's feet and a flat surface should encourage alternate stepping movements. Placing is best elicited by the examiner holding the baby round the top of the trunk in an upright, suspended position. The baby is slowly raised until the dorsum of the foot touches a protruding edge (often the edge of a cot). In response to this stimulus the baby will purposefully flex their hip and knee and lift (or place) the foot on top of the protruding surface.

Abnormal findings

Generally, reflexes that are overly exaggerated or where there is an inability to elicit the required response can indicate the presence of a neurological abnormality. However, one should first check that other factors are not affecting the baby. For example, the baby may be agitated and wanting to feed, or may be affected by maternal drugs (e.g. pethidine) or the aftermath of a traumatic birth. Repeating the neurological assessment when the baby is calm and comfortable would be advantageous.

In the event of any abnormal findings, referral to the senior paediatrician should be expedited and a comprehensive record of the details should be completed within the neonatal record. Parents will need time with the neonatologist in order to discuss the findings and any future investigations that may be required.

36 Common skin conditions

Figure 36.1 (a) Erythema toxicum neonatorum. (b) Harlequin colour change. (c) Cutis marmorata.
Source: Reproduced with permission from Irvine et al. (2011)/John Wiley & Sons.

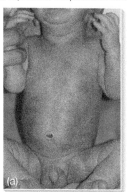
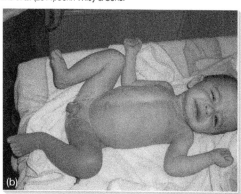
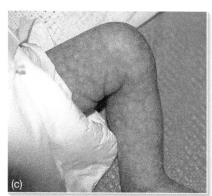

Table 36.1 Common terms used to describe skin conditions.

Erythema	Patches of skin with superficial reddening
Macule	Flat, dark area on the skin
Naevus	Raised birth mark
Papule	Pimple or spot
Pustule	Papule filled with pus
Vesicle	Fluid-filled bubble

Box 36.1 Skin care literature to give a global and national perspective.

Kido, M., Yonezawa, K., Haruna, M. et al. (2024). A global survey on national standard care for newborn bathing. *Japan Journal of Nursing Science* **21**: e12558. https://doi.org/10.1111/jjns.12558
Fleming, S., and Hunter, L. (2021). Newborn skin cleansing practices and their rationales: a systematic review of the literature. Oxford Brookes University. https://radar.brookes.ac.uk/radar/file/a40d4596-d51d-4e44-82f4-efda91730eef/1/Newborn%20skin%20cleansing%20practices%20-%202021%20-%20Fleming%20Hunter.pdf (accessed February 2024).

Table 36.2 Conditions that are commonly seen in neonates.

Condition	Appearance	Management/treatment
Naevus simplex	Occurs in 40% of newborn babies, presenting as poorly defined flat pink macules on the upper eyelid or above the brow line and mid-forehead, or in the hair at the nape of the neck. Although the latter may persist into adulthood, the former tends to fade during the first year. It should not appear elsewhere on the body	No treatment required other than informing the parent(s)
Erythema toxicum neonatorum	Small, firm, white–yellow pustules with an erythematous base, appearing between 1 and 2 days post birth (see Figure 36.1a)	No treatment required and the condition will usually self-resolve within a week of life
Milia	Occurs in 50% of newborn babies, presenting as small (1–2 mm in size), white vesicles, which are mainly filled with sebaceous fluid plus a small quantity of keratin, of 1–2 mm in size on the face or scalp	No treatment required, usually resolves spontaneously after a few weeks
Sebaceous gland hyperplasia	Multiple white and yellow papules, commonly on the cheeks, upper lips and forehead, where sebaceous gland cells are most numerous. Develops as a response to the influence of maternal hormonal influences on the pilosebaceous follicles	No treatment required, usually resolves spontaneously within a few months
Nappy rash	Caused by prolonged exposure to stools and urine, rubbing of nappies, use of soaps or detergents. May occur as a consequence of illness or diarrhoea. The skin in the nappy area may become inflamed and/or develop spots, pustules or blisters	Frequent nappy changes, cleansing from front to back with plain water or newborn baby wipes. Apply barrier cream sparingly. Time spent with area uncovered may also help
Neonatal seborrhoeic dermatitis	'Cradle cap'. Possibly caused by overactive sebaceous glands stimulated by maternal hormones. Presents as inflammation; greasy scales usually form on the scalp and a non-irritating rash may sometimes extend to the face, ears, neck, flexures and nappy area. Milder cases may resolve within a few weeks without treatment. If necessary, frequent shampoos and gently removing the softened scales may help, or applying an emollient overnight before washing the scalp. If it does not demonstrate signs of resolving, refer the baby	An antifungal shampoo and mild topical corticosteroid can be prescribed

The functions of human skin are multifactorial in that if intact it provides a mechanical barrier against micro-organisms and toxins. The thickness of the stratum corneum (the outer layer of the skin) plays an important part in thermoregulation and reducing fluid loss. Communication and learning are enhanced as a result of the sensory input derived from the nerve endings within the dermis.

However, the skin of a newborn baby is immature, alkaline and not yet colonised by the normal fauna and flora that assist in protection against harmful bacteria. During the third trimester of pregnancy, amniotic fluid and vernix (discarded cells from the stratum corneum) raise the acidity of the stratum corneum. The level of vernix on the baby's skin has usually reduced by birth, but as it acts as a natural cleanser and moisturiser, and is an anti-infective and antioxidant, so it is important not to try to remove the vernix from the baby unless it sits in large clumps that will attract dust and dirt. By approximately 5–10 days of age the skin of the term infant has become more acidic and the uppermost layer has become drier and less vulnerable, both of which help to protect the neonate from infection.

Understanding infant skin structure informs practitioner awareness in relation to good skin care practice (Nutfilloyevna et al. 2024). The thickness of the stratum corneum varies depending on the age of the baby, but in a term infant it is only 30% of the depth of that of an adult. This allows for greater permeability, which may not only cause excessive dryness but can also allow for easier absorption of chemicals from creams, lotions or soap (Kelleher et al., 2021). At term, the dermis is only 60% of the depth of that in an adult. Therefore, traumatic delivery or scratches from an amnihook or scalp electrode can cause a breech in the skin barrier through which infection can enter.

Skin care and use of skin preparations

The aim of skin care is to avoid injury and prevent excessive dryness that can cause cracking and fissures, particularly around the wrists, which may lead to infection. Parents should understand the risk associated with using creams and lotions on their baby's skin and should be advised to use plain water for bathing. Current research recommends that no lubricants should be used on neonatal skin as there appears to be a link with a rising level of eczema (Goldsmith et al., 2023). See Box 36.1 for further sources that give insight into global and national perspectives on skin cleansing practices.

Skin problems in neonates are quite common, but most of the time they are benign and will resolve relatively quickly. However, there are some skin conditions and birth marks that can pose a significant risk to health. The role of practitioners is to inspect the neonatal skin regularly and be able to identify the more common neonatal skin conditions and those that warrant medical referral. Parents will often need comprehensive information and discussion, even with those skin conditions that are frequently observed in neonates.

Common skin conditions: birth to 14 days

The conditions and birth marks that appear during the first 2 weeks of life include conditions such as those of a physiological origin, non-infective (often transient), vascular and/or developmental, inheritable and inflammatory conditions. The chapters on neonatal skin focus on the more common conditions that may present themselves during the first 2 weeks. Some of the terms commonly used to describe the appearance of a skin condition can be seen in Table 36.1.

Cysts, papules and vesicles

Practitioners need to appreciate the differing appearance of various skin conditions and their management (Table 36.2).

Erythema toxicum neonatorum is thought to occur as a defensive mechanism, as each papule contains eosinophils that help to allay infection. The papules appear primarily on the face and trunk, each one visible for a few hours and then another appears in a different location (Figure 36.1a). The condition is usually only visible during the time it takes the skin to become more acidic and develop the natural fauna and flora of extrauterine life, approximately 10 days, but occasionally will last up to 2 weeks.

Milia and **sebaceous gland hyperplasia** can be observed in approximately 50% of newborn babies. **Nappy rash** can occur at any time from birth if skin care is neglected. Parents need to be aware that applying a barrier cream may block the absorbency of modern nappies, allowing urine to sit close to the baby's skin rather than being absorbed into the nappy lining. The excoriated skin is also more vulnerable to *Candida albicans*, which should be looked for as both baby and mother (particularly if breastfeeding) may need to be prescribed treatment. By 1 week of age, **seborrhoeic dermatitis** (cradle cap) may also appear, but it often occurs later than 2 weeks post birth.

Epstein pearls may be visible as whitish-yellow, keratin-filled cysts on the neonatal gum or palate. A pearl may also be seen on the tip of the penis or other areas of the male genitalia, where it may be mistaken for a blister of more sinister origin. In both cases these have usually disappeared by the second week of life. A **sucking blister** can often be seen on a baby's hand where it has been suckling in utero. These should be kept clean, but will resolve within a few days.

Atopic dermatitis is a common problem in infancy although it does not usually present until 2–4 months of age. However, if the parents have a family history of eczema, hay fever or asthma, early discussion as to how to reduce possible allergic triggers can have a positive effect on the severity of the condition if it does appear (Kelleher et al., 2021).

Vascular immaturity

Harlequin colour change is seen most frequently in preterm babies and is thought to be a vascular manifestation of the changes that occur in the autonomic system in the newborn. When a baby lies slightly on its side, this condition presents as a marked paleness along the upper part of the body (Figure 36.1b). It can affect 10% of term babies, usually lasting for a few seconds or minutes, but it is transient and without any other anomalies it requires no treatment. Similarly, **acrocyanosis** is a benign condition that can be seen during the first week of life. It is characterised by bluish hands and feet as the neonatal circulation stabilises after birth. It is unaccompanied by other anomalies and usually resolves by 1 week of age. However, prolonged and repeated events should be investigated further and the baby's cardiovascular system assessed for any anomalies.

Cutis marmorata (marbled skin)

Neonates who have cooled may exhibit this condition whereby the skin, particularly on the legs, demonstrates a marbled effect (Figure 36.1c). Some areas of the skin will be vasodilated (look red), whereas others will be vasoconstricted (look pale) because of the immaturity of the nerves linked to superficial capillaries. Assessment of the baby – particularly temperature – should be instigated. As the baby warms the phenomenon will gradually disappear. Why the baby became cold in the first place should be explored, and if the condition is slow to resolve the baby's blood sugar levels should be evaluated and the possibility of infection (in which physiology requires more energy use) should be considered. There is a permanent form of this condition (congenital generalised phlebectasia), but it is rare and will be exacerbated on crying. The condition can also occur in relation to vascular malformation or cutis marmorata telangiectasia, and may persist in trisomy 21 and de Lange syndrome.

37 Atypical skin conditions

Figure 37.1 Congenital dermal melanosis.
Source: Reproduced with permission from Lissauer and Avroy (2011) / John Wiley & Sons.

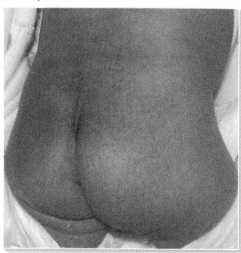

Figure 37.2 Congenital melanocytic naevus.
Source: Reproduced with permission from Lissauer and Avroy (2011) / John Wiley & Sons.

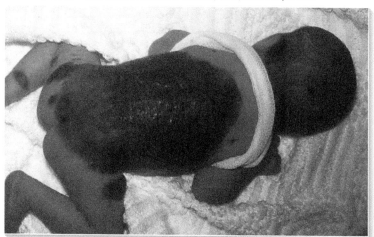

Figure 37.3 Naevus flammeus (Port wine stain).
Source: Reproduced with permission from Lissauer and Avroy (2011) / John Wiley & Sons.

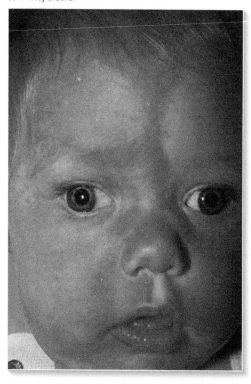

Figure 37.4 Embryonic milk lines.

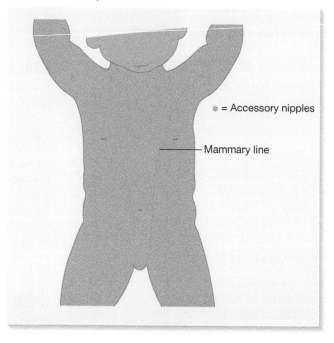

● = Accessory nipples

— Mammary line

Physical Examination of the Newborn at a Glance, Second Edition. Dr Lyn Dolby and Denise (Dee) Campbell.
© 2025 John Wiley & Sons Ltd. Published 2025 by John Wiley & Sons Ltd.

Pigmented birthmarks

Congenital dermal melanosis (hyperpigmented macule) used to be called Mongolian blue spot, but the name was updated to reflect that it is not a birth mark that occurs *only* in those with Mongolian heritage as was perceived when first discovered. Staff need to be mindful that the name was not changed because it was deemed racial, plus that other countries sometimes still refer to the original name or refer to it under the umbrella of 'blue spot' birth marks. It is usually an inherited condition, mainly occurring in Asian, African and African American families, and a smaller percentage will occur in those of Latin American, Caribbean and Spanish heritage, with the remainder in white and mixed-race families. It presents as blue-grey macules or patches (Figure 37.1), commonly over the buttocks, coccyx, thighs, arms and shoulders and much more rarely over the face or front torso. They are caused by a collection of melanocytes infiltrating the dermis, but most will gradually fade over 3–6 years unless they are deeply pigmented.

It is usually a benign, congenital hyperpigmentation, but practitioners need to be aware that it may be indicative of related conditions such as Hurler syndrome, Hunter's syndrome and Niemann-Pick disease. Therefore, it is important to investigate the gene heritage, assess the baby's well-being and consider the depth of pigmentation to ensure timely paediatric referral if necessary. As with other birth marks, the number of macules, size and location must be documented on a body map and the parent(s) informed in case the condition is mistaken for non-accidental injuries when the baby goes home.

Sebaceous naevi (sebaceous nevus of Jadassohn) occur in neonates either at birth or within the first year. They usually appear as elevated, orange-brown granular plaques on the face and/or scalp that develop uniform, wart-like projections. Paediatric referral is required for an expert opinion (Knittel and Ardakani, 2023).

Congenital melanocytic naevus is an uncommon naevus that is visible at birth in neonates and appears as a brown-black area of the skin due to the deep extension of melanocytes into the dermis. It is often flat but can occasionally be hairy (or become hairy over time) or raised (Figure 37.2). The size must be recorded accurately and it has been suggested that any naevus measuring more than 1.5 cm requires referral (Kinsler, 2023) so that the parent(s) receive contemporary guidance and appropriate support. Some newborns present with multiple naevi or with a 'garment' naevus that covers part of the body, which raises concern for malignancy and abnormalities of the CNS.

Capillary vascular malformations

Naevus flammeus (port wine stain) presents at birth as a flat red or purple patch (Figure 37.3) and is caused by a non-inherited, genetic mutation in the embryo. Most often it is sited in head and neck areas (65%), but it does occur in other areas of the body and tends to be unilateral. In time, lesions thicken and become darker. Early referral to a specialist is recommended as lesions in particular areas can signify potential risks: those round the eye increase the risk of glaucoma; lesions on the forehead and scalp may be associated with fitting as in Sturge-Weber syndrome; and soft tissue and bone overgrowth is associated with Klippel-Trenaunay syndrome.

Congenital haemangiomas

These developmental errors of abnormal angiogenesis are common in childhood. There are different categories, with most causing only mild impact, but a few can create more severe issues in relation to the effectiveness of blood volume/flow, breathing difficulties and at times pressure and obstruction of sight. Haemangiomas present in approximately 3% (3 females : 1 male) of the population, with the majority appearing within the first month of life.

Strawberry naevi (infantile superficial haemangioma, capillary haemangioma) is a benign tumour or birth mark consisting of a dense, often raised cluster of blood vessels in the skin, which occurs in 1% of the population. Approximately 20% are present at birth but 90% will appear by 1 month of age. Haemangiomas are the most common infantile tumour, most frequently seen in white female infants and those born prematurely. The lesions grow rapidly (80% in the first month), which can cause bleeding and ulceration, and reach a maximum size at approximately 9 months of age. By 4 years of age they have usually regressed by 80% and 95% of lesions will have almost or completely resolved. However, deep lesions can cause anatomical distortion of underlying structures, for example those lying over the eyes, nose or under the chin can cause amblyopia (reduced vision), breathing difficulties and so on. Therefore, immediate systemic treatment with a beta-blocker (which can be administered topically) is often required to aid in rapid involution of the haemangioma to protect sight and breathing. Other forms of treatment may include laser therapy and systemic corticosteroids.

Pre-auricular nodules and peri-auricular sinuses

Pre-auricular nodules present as unilateral, bilateral or multiple fleshy papules in the pre-auricular area of the ear, but unless accompanied by any signs of a congenital syndrome are often treated later by cosmetic surgery if wished.

Peri-auricular sinuses generally occur in individuals of Asian or African descent (4%) compared with approximately 0.9% in the white population. They can occur bilaterally, but are more commonly seen unilaterally. At present the literature tends to agree that such sinuses do not impact on hearing per se, but there is a possibility for infection and therefore paediatric referral is required.

Supernumerary nipples

Accessory mammary tissue can occur anywhere along the embryologic lines (the 'milk line') that run on each side of the body from the axillae to the inner thighs (Figure 37.4). Accessory nipples can occur anywhere along these lines, but the further away from the breast tissue the less mammary tissue will be present. In neonates, the accessory nipple appears as a tiny, light brown macule. In adulthood, it appears as a small brown papule that protrudes slightly above skin level. In women, if this papule is very close to or on the breast itself and has underlying breast tissue, milk may be produced postnatally.

Neonatal seborrheic dermatitis (cradle cap)

It is thought that this condition occurs as a result of over-active sebaceous glands that are stimulated by the residual maternal hormones in the baby. In mild forms it appears as scaly patches on the scalp, which will often resolve within a few weeks without needing treatment other than frequent washing of the scalp with shampoo and gently removing any loose, softened scales. However, it can appear as a thick crusting, resembling white or yellow scales, which may require the use of an emollient. At times the condition may continue, for which an antifungal shampoo and/or mild topical corticosteroid can be prescribed.

38 Head

Figure 38.1 (a, b) Newborn skull showing bones, suture lines and fontanelles.

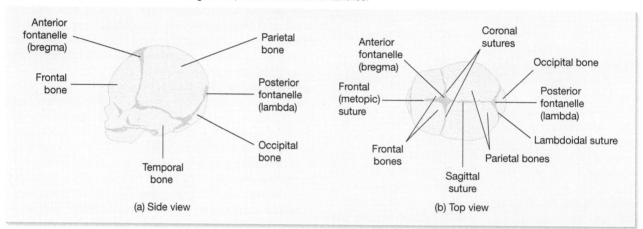

(a) Side view

(b) Top view

Figure 38.2 Measuring the anterior fontanelle.

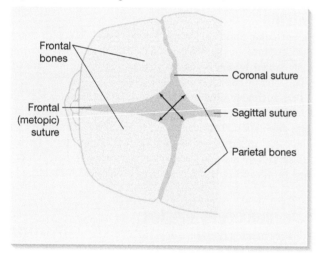

Figure 38.3 Caput succedaneum or cephalhaematoma.

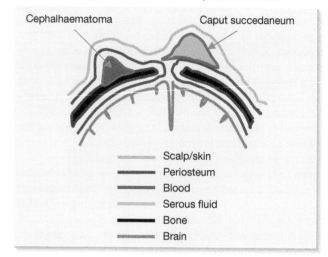

Scalp/skin
Periosteum
Blood
Serous fluid
Bone
Brain

Figure 38.4 (a–c) Moulding related to positions and presentations.
Source: Brosansky et al. (2021), Zittelli and Davis' Atlas of Pediatric Diagnosis, 2012.

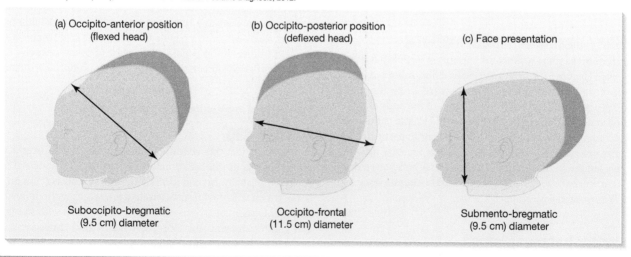

(a) Occipito-anterior position (flexed head)

Suboccipito-bregmatic (9.5 cm) diameter

(b) Occipito-posterior position (deflexed head)

Occipito-frontal (11.5 cm) diameter

(c) Face presentation

Submento-bregmatic (9.5 cm) diameter

This chapter considers the examination of the vault of the skull and scalp, including inspection and palpation of the seven bones, suture lines and fontanelles (Figures 38.1 and 38.2). The practitioner is looking for signs of trauma, excessive moulding, swelling, ridges, decompressions, unusual diameters, bulging or sunken fontanelles, birth marks, lesions or abnormal head circumference measurement.

Head circumference

The head circumference (occipito-frontal circumference) indirectly measures the brain, cerebral fluids and skull. At term, for boys this is in the range of 33.1–35.8 cm (15–85th centiles with a 50th centile of 34.5 cm); for girls, 32.7–35.8 cm (15–85th centiles with a 50th centile of 33.9 cm) (WHO, 2024). This measurement can be affected by pathological abnormalities, but typically will be altered by harmless oedema, haematoma or moulding (Figures 38.3 and 38.4). Measure the widest diameter to include the occipital and frontal prominences (1–2 cm above the glabella) using a disposable, non-stretchable tape. Take three measurements (to the nearest millimetre) and record the largest of these.

Head shape and moulding

Moulding is a normal process resulting from the movement of the skull bones when compressed before or during labour. The skull bones bend slightly and overlap partially (at suture lines and fontanelles) to reduce the diameters of the head and facilitate delivery. Diameters under pressure reduce by up to 1 cm, while those without pressure elongate. The degree and direction of moulding relate to fetal positioning and the pressure experienced (Figure 38.4). Moulding is harmless unless it is excessive or rapid, or if decompression occurs too rapidly.

The head shape can be significantly affected by fetal presentation antenatally, type of delivery, length of labour, maternal pelvic shape and presentation and position of the fetus during labour and delivery. For example, the breech presentation infant delivered by caesarean section will have a round-shaped head that has never experienced any prolonged pressure, whereas the deflexed head of an occipito-posterior position will experience upward moulding along the submento-bregmatic diameter (Figure 38.4).

Excessive moulding

This occurs in a term infant when there is either an abnormal head or excessive pressure during labour or delivery, for instance with dystocia or an instrumental delivery. This excessive moulding may damage the bones (through excessive bending) or intracranial membranes, vessels or tissues. Excessive moulding is a particular risk for the softer skull of the premature infant.

Fontanelles

There are six fontanelles (Figure 38.1). The two sphenoid and two mastoid fontanelles only show with increased intracranial pressure. The two main fontanelles are the rhomboid or kite-shaped anterior fontanelle (bregma), where the frontal (metopic), coronal and sagittal sutures meet; and the triangular, posterior fontanelle (lambda), where the sagittal and lambdoidal sutures meet. Inspection and palpation must be carried out on a quiet, calm newborn as crying will tense the fontanelles. Assess for size, swelling, decompression, tenseness, bulging or sunken appearance. If unsure, re-examine with the newborn in a sitting position.

The size is measured diagonally, from bone to bone in both directions (Figure 38.2). The two results are added together and divided by two. The bregma is 0.6–3.6 cm (average 2 cm) and can take between 6 and 24 months to close (average 14 months). The lambda is smaller at 0.3–1.5 cm (average 0.6 cm) and typically closes by 2 months. An enlarged bregma (or delayed closure) may be associated with hypothyroidism, achondroplasia (dwarfism), trisomy 21 (Down syndrome), rickets or increased intracranial pressure. A small bregma may indicate microcephaly. A third fontanelle, between the anterior and posterior fontanelles, may be associated with hypothyroidism and trisomy 21. Bulging fontanelles may be associated with intracranial pressure, hydrocephalus, inflammation (encephalitis), hypoxia, trauma, tumour (scalp or intracranial), heart disease or metabolic disorders. A sunken fontanelle is associated with dehydration.

Common abnormalities

- **Abrasions or lacerations of the scalp**: caused by interventions (amnihook, scalp electrode, fetal blood sampling, instrumental delivery, operative delivery); resolve spontaneously.
- **Aplasia cutis congenita**: typically 1 cm wide, hairless, scalp lesion in front of the lambda. Can be flat, keloid, blistery or ulcerated with possible exudate. Rarely associated with an underlying defect. Most resolve but leave a bald patch.
- **Asynclitism**: asymmetry of the head resulting from uneven pressure on a tilted head during labour. Resolves spontaneously without problems.
- **Caput succedaneum** (Figure 38.3): oedema of the presenting part caused by cervical pressure or vacuum extraction. Present from birth, pits with pressure and crosses suture lines. Resolves within days.
- **Cephalhaematoma** (Figure 38.3): blood between the periosteum and bone so does not cross suture lines. May be present at birth or develop in the very early post-natal period. Typically these are harmless and gradually reduce over a period of 4–6 weeks, but they may take months to go. In rare circumstances they may lie over a fracture or may calcify (harden) and not reduce.
- **Craniosynostosis**: premature closing or fusing of a suture. Limits growth in the area fused so causes uneven head shape. Associated with rickets, hyperthyroidism and numerous syndromes.
- **Fracture**: usually linear, may be depressed. Rarely leaks cerebrospinal fluid via nose or ear (requires antibiotics). Depressed fractures may require surgery but most fractures heal without problems.
- **Hair**: low hairline, increased quantity of hair or brittleness are more common with congenital abnormalities.
- **Hydrocephalus**: increased cerebrospinal fluid.
- **Macrocephaly**: head circumference above 90th centile.
- **Microcephaly**: head circumference below 10th centile.
- **Subgaleal (subaponeurotic) haemorrhage**: appearance of scalp oedema but contains blood. Present at birth, increases and spreads, resolves over 2–3 weeks. In rare cases massive haemorrhage, shock and death.
- **Tumour**: extracranial or intracranial.
- **Vascular skin lesions (birth mark)**: multiple visible haemangiomas require investigation of possible occurrence on internal organs too.
- **Whorls**: hair follicles slope with skin stretch linked to growth of head. More than two whorls, or any over the parietal region, may be linked to abnormal brain growth.

39 Facies

Figure 39.1 Asymmetry when crying.
Source: Lissauer et al. (2020)/John Wiley & Sons.

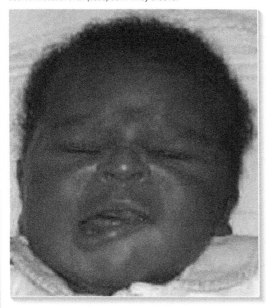

Figure 39.2 Normal ear position.

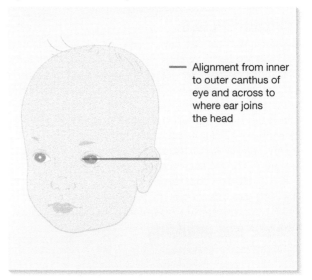

— Alignment from inner to outer canthus of eye and across to where ear joins the head

Figure 39.3 Normal eye position.

Eyes equidistant from midline of face.
Inner canthus aligned to edge of nose.
Space between eyes same as eye width

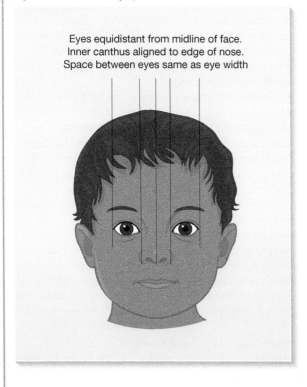

Figure 39.4 Facial palsy.
Source: Lissauer et al. (2020)/John Wiley & Sons.

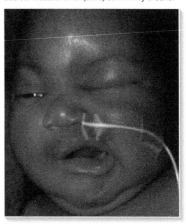

Figure 39.5 Normal external ear.

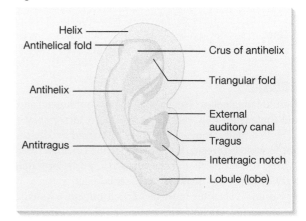

Helix
Antihelical fold
Crus of antihelix
Triangular fold
Antihelix
External auditory canal
Tragus
Antitragus
Intertragic notch
Lobule (lobe)

Physical Examination of the Newborn at a Glance, Second Edition. Dr Lyn Dolby and Denise (Dee) Campbell.
© 2025 John Wiley & Sons Ltd. Published 2025 by John Wiley & Sons Ltd.

This chapter considers the facial characteristics including the nose and extending to the ears. The eyes and mouth have their own more detailed chapters to enhance the information contained here. Whenever possible, following a review of the family history, it is advisable to begin by paying attention to the facial features of the parent(s). This will often explain idiosyncrasies in the features observed on the newborn – they may be familial inheritances.

Asymmetry and dysmorphia

Assessment of facial symmetry and dysmorphia should take place while the newborn is quiet as well as during crying. Look for any lack of uniformity across the two halves of the face (Figure 39.1); depression of the jaw (micrognathia – may be associated with Pierre-Robin syndrome); abnormality in shape, size, structure or positioning of individual features; or the occurrence of any unexpected aspect. The eyes should be the same size and equidistant from the midline of the nose, with the inner aspect of the eyes aligning with the outer width of the nose (Figures 39.2 and 39.3). There should be approximately one eye distance between the two eyes. Orbital hypotelorism and hypertelorism are the names given to eyes that are too close or too widely spaced apart, respectively. If a problem is identified, an opinion is needed on whether this is a temporary issue (positional pressure in utero or delivery trauma), a deformity or evidence of a syndrome or chromosomal abnormality. Observation during crying aids in identification of reduced or absent movements and this includes drooping of the mouth and loss of forehead wrinkles, for example facial palsy (Figure 39.4), or a more permanent paralysis (linked to the seventh cranial nerve).

Skin

The facial skin is inspected for evidence of bruising, trauma, cyanosis, jaundice, birth marks, tumours or spots. The most common causes of trauma link to the presentation and type of delivery. A face or brow presentation and associated pressure from the cervix or forceps application can cause significant trauma. The degree and placement of any trauma must be documented very accurately to monitor improvements or worsening and to prevent allegations of abuse. Discolouration of the skin and dysmorphia can result from any birth mark, but particularly haemangiomas where the tumour develops over or is attached to a facial feature.

The skin colour can also be affected by jaundice and resultant yellowing of the face and sclera. Harlequin syndrome can extend to the face – a phenomenon where redness, because of increased peripheral blood supply, occurs on one side of the body (often the lowermost side) while reduced pigmentation and pallor occur on the opposite (and often uppermost) side. Circumoral cyanosis (blue discolouration around the mouth only) may be a normal presentation in the first 24 hours after birth. Similarly, a mild red to purplish colouration during crying can be associated with polycythaemia and this will resolve as the newborn's high haemoglobin level resolves. Any generalised cyanosis, spreading to the body, needs further investigation of full airway patency, pulmonary disease, sepsis or neurological concerns.

Lesions, spots, pustules and blisters occur commonly on the face. These must be identified to inform and reassure parents plus to advise management as appropriate. The most commonly identified are the benign erythema toxicum and milia.

Nose

The nose is examined for its appearance, site, symmetry (to the midline), shape, patency, lesions, secretions and for signs of excessive sneezing. There are a wide range of normal shapes but many syndromes may affect the nose. A flattened or low bridge may be associated with trisomy 21 (Down syndrome) or FAS and a short, broad nose may be associated with Noonan syndrome or FAS.

Newborns are nose breathers when at rest but mouth breathers when crying. Hence, cyanosis apparent when the newborn is resting that clears during crying may indicate nasal blockage. The most common blockage is choanal atresia, which will not be visible, but a deviated septum, narrowing or absence of the nostrils, lesions or external malformation of the nose should be looked for. In cases of partial blockage, nasal flare may be evident as a result of greater effort required to nose breathe.

Newborn nasal secretions are minimal and either clear or slightly frothy (linked to the clearing of amniotic fluid). Yellow secretions occur during pulmonary infection and thick, white discharges can indicate viral inflammation. Heavily frothy discharge may be seen with oesophageal atresia. Nasal congestion is rare at birth but may be present by 6 weeks. It is more commonly associated with inflammation and allergy caused by dry air or irritants than with infection. Sneezing is generally normal but when excessive can indicate drug withdrawal and neonatal abstinence syndrome.

Philtrum

Long, indistinct, absent or deeper than normal grooves below the nose to the upper lip can all be associated with chromosomal abnormalities and syndromes such as Prader-Willi, Noonan and FAS. Broader than average grooves may be seen in autism spectrum conditions.

External ear (auricle or pinna)

Ears are examined for shape, site, symmetry (to the face and each other), attachment, lesions and structural abnormality. Patency is covered by the hearing tests, but signs of atresia are also assessed. Anotia is the term given to absence of an external ear; microtia is associated with an abnormally small ear (often malformed); and macrotia is an enlarged ear (often otherwise normal but sometimes linked to problems such as haemangiomas). The ear should be well formed (Figure 39.5) with the upper margin aligned with the inner and outer canthus of the eye (Figure 39.2). Some initial swelling or squashing of the ear may be positional or a result of delivery, but the cartilage should recoil easily to a normal position.

Thickening of the outer or inner aspect of the helix, at the point where the top third begins (Darwinian tubercules), is common but rarely significant. Hairy ears may be familial, relate to a syndrome or link to maternal diabetes mellitus. Clefts, grooves, dimples, pits, skin tags, sinuses and fistulae may be abnormalities of aesthetic concern only or may contain cartilage, cysts or tumours and be associated with deafness or a syndrome. Malformed, abnormally attached or low-set ears may also link to chromosomal or urogenital abnormality and deafness (e.g. trisomy 17 or 18; Noonan syndrome).

40 Eyes

Figure 40.1 (a) Common form of coloboma; (b) fundal (red eye) reflex; (c) congenital cataract.
Source: Reproduced with permission from Lissauer and Fanaroff (2011) / John Wiley & Sons.

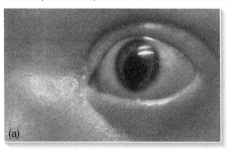 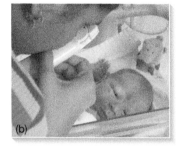 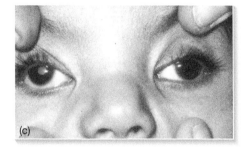

(a)   (b)   (c)

Table 40.1 Risk factors for congenital cataract.

Risk factor	Comments
Congenital cataract (*prime risk factor*)	First-degree relative with a family history of bilateral congenital cataract or resulting from a hereditary autosomal dominant condition
Low birth weight	Birth weight <1500 g
Low gestational age	<32 weeks' gestation May be caused by trauma rather than prematurity per se
Family history	First-degree relative with a congenital ocular condition or one that developed in early childhood, e.g. aniridia, coloboma, glaucoma or retinoblastoma
Maternal infection	Congenital rubella syndrome Toxoplasmosis Cytomegalovirus
Genetic syndrome	For example, in trisomy 21 5–10% of babies will have cataracts at birth. Differences in risk reporting are due to the provision of a result from the specific sample group from which the data was collected, thus other literature from a different source will state >50% Continued reassessment required
Galactosaemia	Caused by changes in the metabolism of carbohydrates and an excess of sugar in the blood and aqueous humour disrupting normal development
Idiopathic	50% will have no identifiable cause

Table 40.2 Examination findings (all to be documented within neonatal record, PCHR and S4N).

Screen negative	No anomalies found: • Parent(s) to be informed of signs that may indicate changes to eye status • Next assessment at GP in 6–8 weeks and if normal at this point child will enter Healthy Child Programme **Note:** Babies with no anomaly detected but a history of bilateral congenital or hereditary cataracts in a first-degree relative are at risk of developing early cataracts and may be referred for early specialist opinion in accordance with local NHS Trust protocol
Screen positive	The absence or presence of a partial reflex in one or both eyes Urgent referral to ophthalmologist by **2 weeks** of age Significant concerns should prompt a discussion with ophthalmology service prior to discharge Surgery for severe cataract is often undertaken between 6 and 10 weeks of age for optimal visual outcome
Screen positive at 6 to 8 week infant examination	Baby will be referred as above to be seen by **11 weeks** of age
Information for parent(s) as to when to seek advice	• Baby does not fully open their eyes or eyelid opening is asymmetrical • Deterioration of visual interest, e.g. does not fixate or follow object or light source • Baby's eyes look unusual • Wobbling (nystagmus) of the eyes, consistent eye misalignment • White reflex consistently seen on flash photography • One eye demonstrates a lack of or asymmetry of 'red eye' on flash photography

Physical Examination of the Newborn at a Glance, Second Edition. Dr Lyn Dolby and Denise (Dee) Campbell.
© 2025 John Wiley & Sons Ltd. Published 2025 by John Wiley & Sons Ltd.

In the United Kingdom, approximately 2–3/10,000 babies (200 per year in England) are born each year with a congenital cataract and in 50% both eyes will be affected. Only 40 of these babies will have a family history of the condition. Cataracts account for the highest treatable cause of blindness in the United Kingdom and worldwide. Therefore, early detection and treatment for congenital cataract(s) are paramount if the child is to achieve the optimum possible visual acuity. However, the presence of other ocular conditions that disrupt light from entering the eye or disrupt the ocular pathways also needs to be detected early to prevent similar disruption to visual pathway development that is occurring in these critical early weeks of life. Local NHS Trust guidance needs to be followed in the presence of risk factors or other eye abnormalities.

Formation of the eye

Formation of the eye commences at approximately 22 days post conception. By the third trimester, the fetus can detect bright light. At birth, a baby can see objects up to 25 cm away (the approximate distance from the mother's face to the baby while feeding). Babies are attracted by highly contrasting patterns of black and white or primary colours. A baby should be able to fixate on an object, with a particular preference for faces, and begin to follow it even when a couple of hours old, although the macula is poorly developed at birth so precise fixation is not possible. However, any ocular condition that interferes with fixation and ocular stimulation can delay or reduce the ability to develop binocular vision (Box 40.1) and with social interaction or parental bonding.

Eye examination

The eye examination aspect of the NIPE should follow the PHE newborn eye screening guidance (PHE, 2021d). Prior to physical examination, the maternity records should always be reviewed for the presence of risk factors (Table 40.1). The parent(s) should also be asked if there is any family history of eye disorders in childhood and the purpose of the examination should be explained and agreement sought and recorded. It should be noted whether the eyes have been seen since the baby was born, as a very small proportion of babies are born without one eye (anophthalmia) and, even rarer still, an absence of both eyes.

The examination is best carried out when the baby is calm and alert and therefore an opportunistic assessment at any point during the NIPE is preferable. If the baby is reluctant to open their eyes, they should **not** be forced open as trauma can occur to the soft tissue and infection can be introduced. It may help encourage the baby to open their eyes to carry out the examination in a darkened room, holding the baby over the parent's shoulder or raising and lowering the shoulders of the baby while in the supine position to take advantage of the 'doll's eye reflex'.

The examination should be undertaken using an 'outward-in' approach, whereby the outer aspects of the eye are examined first. The size, shape and alignment of the eyes should be noted, with the width of one of the baby's eyes corresponding to the distance between the two eyes. The soft tissue surrounding the eye may be oedematous as a result of pressure against the bony pelvis, but this will resolve during the next 24 hours, but drooping of the eyelid should be documented and the baby referred to a paediatrician as this may be linked to nerve trauma. Similarly, trauma across the eye caused by forceps blades should be noted and if the practitioner has concerns regarding the impact/severity of the trauma the baby must be referred to a senior paediatrician. Eye lashes should sweep outwards as inward-facing lashes can cause corneal scarring. There should be no signs of infection or conjunctivitis, which presents as a sticky discharge with accompanying redness. The most common causes of infection are chlamydia, gonococcal or HSV infection. A severe and/or untreated infection can lead to scarring of the cornea, causing loss of clarity of sight later.

The position, shape, structure and condition of the iris should be noted. A small number of babies have aniridia (absence of the iris or where it has not formed properly) or colobomata. A coloboma (Figure 40.1a) can be recognised by the notch or gap seen within the iris, which in itself usually poses no problem for the developing baby. However, the malformation may extend deeper into the ocular structure and not only affect the underlying structures of the eye, but also the external structures such as the eyelid. It can occur in isolation, but can also appear with other abnormal neonatal features.

An ophthalmoscope (using the large, round, white light setting) should be used to shine the light into the baby's eyes from an approximate distance of 30 cm. Practitioners can also use an 'arc light', which is less costly than a traditional ophthalmoscope, but the key principle remains: the practitioner should take time to visualise the roundness of the pupil and the reflex elicited – this is a time for patience to be employed! Also, research is ongoing in relation to the effectiveness of a digital camera that can provide an 'infrared-reflex image', which may prove to be a more efficient method of screening in the future.

The ability of the baby to fixate on the light and follow it should be assessed. If there is no obstruction to the passage of light, the beam will bounce off the back of the eyeball towards the front of the eye, eliciting what is termed the 'fundal or red reflex' (Figure 40.1b). The red eye that is sometimes seen in photographs depicts exactly the same response, but the colour may be paler or more cream coloured with darker-skinned babies. For this reason, some ophthalmologists prefer using the term 'fundal reflex', with the aim of correcting perception to expect a colour that is appropriate for darker skin tones. It should be noted that the presence of cataracts, glaucoma and retinoblastoma will produce a different response.

Congenital cataract

The early detection of congenital cataracts is the prime reason for conducting the neonatal eye examination. The main risk factor to be noted is a family history of congenital or hereditary cataracts (first-degree relative); other additional factors include low birth weight, low gestational age, trisomy 21, family history of any childhood eye disorder and antenatal exposure to viruses (Table 40.1). If the cataract is fully developed, it may be seen in daylight as a cloudy, silvery disc across the pupil and no red reflex can be elicited when using the ophthalmoscope (Figure 40.1c). Immediate referral to the paediatric team is required, with expert referral required within 2 weeks of detection.

Retinoblastoma

This is the most common intraocular tumour to be found in childhood and is a malignant tumour arising from the cells within the retina. Commonly, only a white (leukocoria) reflex can be elicited. Occasionally, later detection may be accompanied by strabismus (squint). The seriousness of this condition should not be under-estimated and immediate referral to an ophthalmologist is necessary, as the condition can be life-threatening. The emotional impact on the parents is considerable.

Glaucoma

This condition may at first be suspected because of the presence of a watery eye, which may be mistaken for obstruction of the lacrimal duct that drains excess moisture (lubrication) away from the eye. Infantile glaucoma is usually accompanied by a large and cloudy cornea and photophobia. The usual cause is a blockage preventing the drainage of intraocular fluid, leading to a rise in intraocular pressure and enlargement of the globe of the eye with accompanying pressure to the optic nerve. Again, prompt referral to an ophthalmologist is paramount.

Examination findings and documentation

The examination findings should be clearly documented, including the actions taken in the event of a screen positive outcome

(Table 40.2). As with many aspects of the examination of the newborn, parents will need emotional support in the event of abnormal findings. Sensitively informing the parent(s) of the nature of the findings and prompt referral to the paediatric team are paramount.

Information for parents

Discussion with the parent(s) should not only include the findings of the examination, but should also raise their awareness as to when to contact their midwife, GP or health visitor in the event of future concern (Table 40.2). However, parents are sometimes unaware of their baby's ability to fixate, follow an object, and blink soon after birth or why the immaturity of the eye muscles can produce a normal transitory 'squint' appearance in their baby. They should be informed about how far their baby can see, that babies prefer and see in black and white at this age and that they focus intently on an object or person when they are in learning mode and love being talked to – all of which assist in their mental development and strengthen their vision.

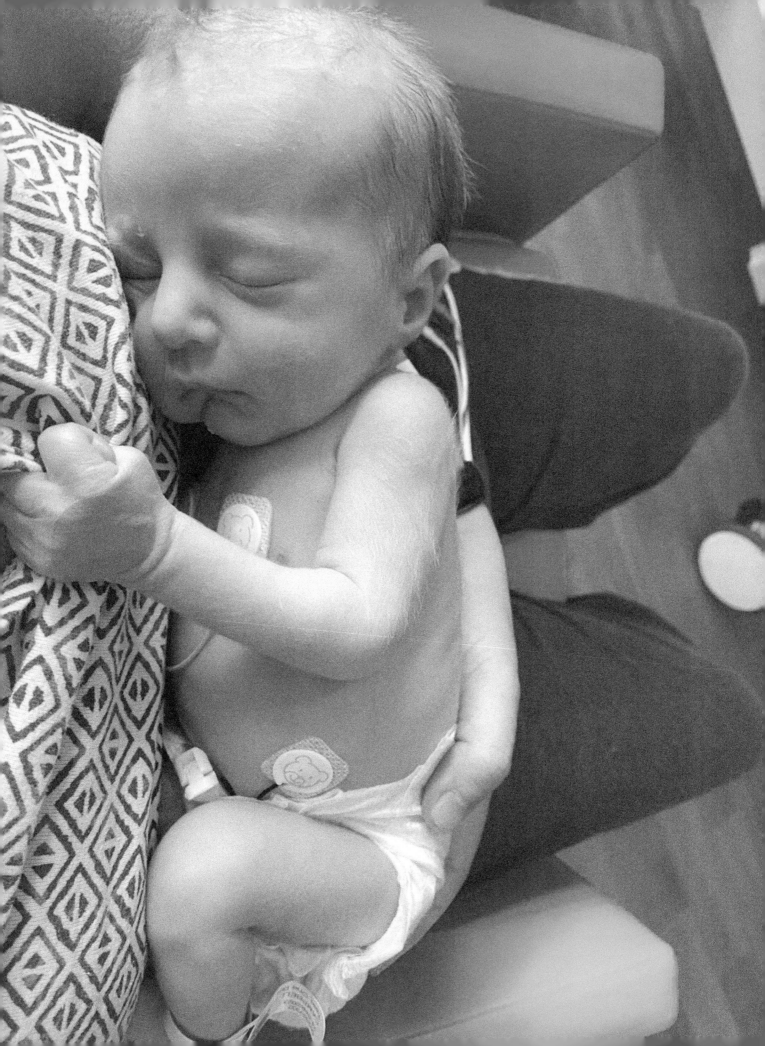

41 Mouth

Figure 41.1 Anatomy of the mouth, indicating the concerns to identify.

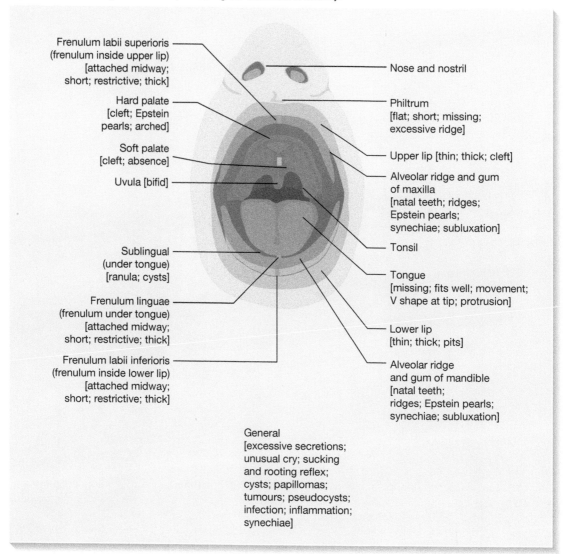

Frenulum labii superioris
(frenulum inside upper lip)
[attached midway;
short; restrictive; thick]

Hard palate
[cleft; Epstein
pearls; arched]

Soft palate
[cleft; absence]

Uvula [bifid]

Sublingual
(under tongue)
[ranula; cysts]

Frenulum linguae
(frenulum under tongue)
[attached midway;
short; restrictive; thick]

Frenulum labii inferioris
(frenulum inside lower lip)
[attached midway;
short; restrictive; thick]

Nose and nostril

Philtrum
[flat; short; missing;
excessive ridge]

Upper lip [thin; thick; cleft]

Alveolar ridge and gum
of maxilla
[natal teeth; ridges;
Epstein pearls;
synechiae; subluxation]

Tonsil

Tongue
[missing; fits well; movement;
V shape at tip; protrusion]

Lower lip
[thin; thick; pits]

Alveolar ridge
and gum of mandible
[natal teeth;
ridges; Epstein pearls;
synechiae; subluxation]

General
[excessive secretions;
unusual cry; sucking
and rooting reflex;
cysts; papillomas;
tumours; pseudocysts;
infection; inflammation;
synechiae]

Figure 41.2 (a–d) Types of cleft lip and palate.
Source: Lissauer et al. (2020) / John Wiley & Sons.

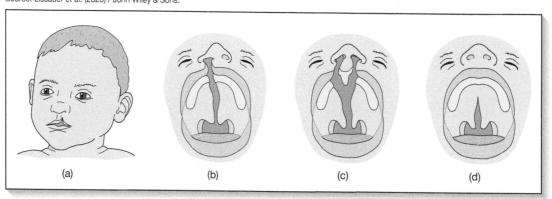

(a)　　　　(b)　　　　(c)　　　　(d)

Physical Examination of the Newborn at a Glance, Second Edition. Dr Lyn Dolby and Denise (Dee) Campbell.
© 2025 John Wiley & Sons Ltd. Published 2025 by John Wiley & Sons Ltd.

This chapter considers examination of the mouth, to include the lips, frenulae, palates, tongue, alveolar ridges and gums (Figure 41.1). The mouth is also relevant to the examination of the newborn reflexes (sucking and rooting), feeding and airway management chapters.

General congenital abnormalities

• **Gingival cysts (dental lamina cysts)** (Diaz de Ortiz and Mendez, 2023) have an epithelial lining and are keratin filled. They are benign, typically painless, sterile and less than 2.5 cm in diameter. Found on the alveolar ridge and more common on the maxilla than the mandible, they disappear within 3–6 months.

• **Palatal cysts (Epstein pearls [EPs] and Bohn's nodules [BNs])** (Diaz de Ortiz and Mendez, 2023) are both benign, 1–3 mm wide, firm papules. EPs are whitish-yellow and found on the mid-palate or gum line, occurring when epithelial tissue is trapped during palate development. BNs are smooth and white, found either where the hard and soft palate meet or where the gum joins the lip, and are believed to be remnants of developing salivary glands. They can be solitary but more commonly occur in groups, disappearing by 2–3 weeks of age.

• **Excessive oral secretions and drooling** occur when a newborn has a poor swallow reflex or in conjunction with oesophageal atresia and tracheoesophageal fistula. They can also appear as a secondary symptom of any condition affecting swallowing (e.g. cysts, tumours and macroglossia).

• **Micrognathia** is a small, underdeveloped mandible that can be associated with cleft palate and a number of syndromes, e.g. Pierre-Robin syndrome. When severe the prolapsed tongue restricts or obstructs airways.

• **Retrognathia** is an abnormal position of the maxilla or mandible.

• **Pierre-Robin syndrome** is a combination of micrognathia or retrognathia, cleft palate (U shaped) (Figure 41.2) and glossoptosis, which may partially or fully obstruct the airway. Natal teeth may be present.

• **Subluxation of the jaw** is when the upper and lower jaws are not parallel with each other. The lower jaw (mandible) has partially dislocated with one side pushed back. A fetal malposition has resulted in uneven pressure on the jaw, limiting its movement and causing underdeveloped muscles at the hinge joint.

• **Synechia (oral)** is intermittent adhesions between the lower and upper mouth, restricting opening. They may be epithelial or connective tissue alone, or contain muscle and bone, and may be:
  • Between mandible and maxilla (**syngnathia**), linking the two alveolar ridges.
  • Between tongue and palate (**glossopalatal ankylosis**).
  • Between floor of the mouth and the palate (subglossopalatal membrane).
  • Continuous along the alveolar ridges (fibrous syngnathia).

• **Tumours** may be benign, but when malignant they are associated with a poor survival rate, so early detection and treatment (surgery, chemotherapy and radiation) are essential (Khanmohammadi et al., 2018).

Lips

• **Thin upper lip** may be familial, but consider FAS if smooth philtrum and short palpebral fissures are seen.

• **Cleft lip** (cheiloschisis) (Figure 41.2) occurs unilaterally, bilaterally or in the midline. May be associated with cleft palate; may be complete (extending to nose) or incomplete (indentation or grove); and has increased incidence associated with maternal smoking,

diabetes and epilepsy medication (Centers for Disease Control and Prevention, 2024).

• **Macroschelia** (enlarged lip) may be as a result of tumours or partial or complete double lip (horizontal fold and secondary lip).

• **Microstomia** (small width) is often associated with micrognathia.

• **Macrostomia** (large width) can be unilateral or bilateral; a transverse cleft extends the side of the mouth across the face.

• **Indentations** are rare, but pits, fistulas and sinuses sometimes occur.

Frenula

Each of the frenulae should attach midway. They should not appear thick or prominent, nor should they abnormally limit movement of the anatomy in close proximity. The most common problem identified is tongue tie (ankyloglossia) associated with the frenulum lingae; the tongue tip may be pulled into a V shape with limited extension. Failure to correct the problem through frenuloplasty results in poor latch and nipple pain during breastfeeding, and later speech impediment.

Alveolar ridge and gums

Teeth may be present at birth (natal) or emerge in the first month (neonatal), most commonly lower incisors. Removal is avoided to prevent damage to normal tooth development. If a tooth is mobile (they rarely have firm roots), the risk of trauma or inhalation may necessitate removal. These should be differentiated from EPs.

Hard and soft palate, including uvula

Examination must be both digitally and by visualising with a torch.

• **High-arched palate**: check for craniostenosis and choanal atresia.

• **Bifid uvula**: associated with cleft palate.

• **Cleft palate** (Figure 41.2) (Phalke and Goldman, 2023): this is when the palate at the roof of the mouth fails to fully close during development and a gap (cleft) occurs. It may involve hard and/or soft palate and the alveolar ridge. It is more commonly unilateral, but can be bilateral and may extend into a cleft lip. Cleft palate has a familial association, plus 16% will occur alongside other abnormalities and 7% will be part of a syndrome. Incidence is 1 : 650–1000 live births. Symptoms may include respiratory distress, reflux, prolonged feeds, infant fatigue and inadequate latch.

Tongue

Abnormalities of the tongue are commonly associated with metabolic, endocrine or chromosomal abnormalities and tumours.

• **Aglossia**: absence of or poorly developed tongue.

• **Macroglossia**: a large tongue protruding beyond the alveolar ridge (consider hypothyroidism, trisomy 21 and Beckwith-Wiedemann syndrome).

• **Hypoglossia**: short, incompletely developed tongue.

• **Microglossia**: small tongue.

• **Ranula**: translucent, bluish, mucus cyst under the tongue or in the salivary gland; resolves spontaneously.

• **Glossoptosis**: displacement back into the pharynx with partial or complete airway obstruction; may be due to micrognathia and PRS.

• **Dimples, indentations, nodules, grooves and clefts.**

• **Lingual thyroid**: thyroid gland tissue that has incompletely descended and instead enlarges the back of the tongue.

• **Glossitis**: infection may be present (e.g. oral candida or thrush).

42 Neck and clavicles

Figure 42.1 Newborn with cystic hygroma.
Source: Timothy Joseph Wood/Wikimedia Commons/CC BY SA 4.0.

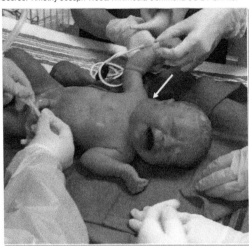

Figure 42.2 Webbing and skin folds.

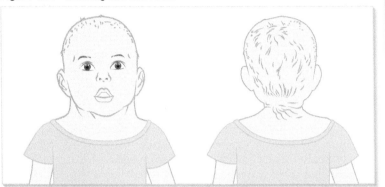

Figure 42.3 Skeleton indicating clavicles.

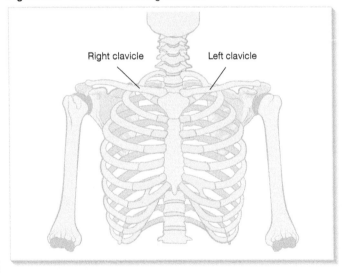

Right clavicle   Left clavicle

Figure 42.4 X-ray multiple fracture left clavicle.
Source: Harlie Raethel / Unsplash.

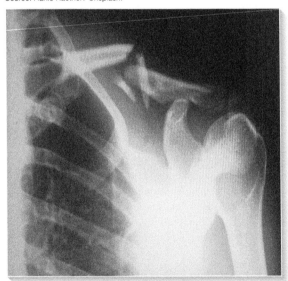

Neck

Inspection must include back, front, all creases and up under the chin. This aims to determine the length of the neck, mobility, flexion, symmetry and the presence of any abnormalities. The neck should enable a rotation of the head by 80° to left and right, lateral flexion by 40°, anterior flexion that allows the chin to almost reach the chest and posterior extension such that the occiput can almost touch the back of the neck. The most common abnormalities detected are the salmon patch (stork mark) and rashes. Otherwise the following abnormalities are all very rare and congenital masses are almost always benign. The most important complications to be aware of are the risks to airway and possibility of a syndrome.

- **Cervical teratoma**: rare masses, solid or cystic, typically benign, unilateral, large (up to 12 cm) and likely to cause airway and/or oesophageal compression. Skin is loose over them.
- **Cystic hygroma** (Figure 42.1) (Auerbach et al., 2023): a benign watery tumour caused by a congenital malformation in the lymphatic drainage system. While rare, it is the most common cervical cystic mass and typically occurs on the left, posterior triangle of the neck; it may also occur bilaterally and in the axilla, thoracic or inguinal areas.

  If it is asymptomatic no immediate treatment is required. Rarely it may require aspiration (decompression) or surgery (to reduce airway obstruction). Transillumination can confirm there is no solid mass and magnetic resonance imaging determines the extent of the cyst. A cystic hygroma can be associated with a short neck and chromosomal abnormality, e.g. Turner syndrome, Klippel-Feil, trisomy 21.
- **Fistulae or sinuses**: rare but may occur in skin folds, so it is important to visualise the whole neck. First appearance may be of a dimple, but examination may determine a deeper fistula or sinus.
- **Goitre**: rare, anterior, midline mass, caused by poor development of thyroid gland and hypothyroidism or maternal medication for hyperthyroidism. Requires hormone replacement therapy.
- **Haemangioma**: these birth marks mostly occur in the head and neck region.
- **Rashes**: the most common inflammatory condition on the neck is miliaria (heat rash). (Rule out meningitis – ensure no unusual cry, sickness, irritability, floppiness or pyrexia.)
- **Low posterior hairline**: a number of syndromes are associated with hair growth low on the back of the neck (e.g. Turner, Noonan and Cornelia de Lange).
- **Salmon patch (angel kiss and stork bite/mark)**: a common group of birth marks involving dilated capillaries at the nape of the neck, eyelids and centre of the forehead.
- **Shortened neck**: a number of syndromes are associated with a short neck (e.g. Turner), with some specifically related to abnormalities of the cervical vertebrae (e.g. Klippel-Feil). The head should still have full rotation.
- **Sternomastoid tumour**: muscle damage involving painless, benign swelling within muscle. Can be caused by traction during delivery or intrauterine positioning, affecting blood supply to the muscle. Resolves spontaneously but may be associated with a fracture too.
- **Torticollis**: restricted movement where a contracted sternomastoid muscle causes the neck to twist or the head to tilt, with chin pointing away from the affected side. It can be related to fetal positioning or instrumental delivery and may be present at birth (congenital) or develop over the first weeks of life. It is painless and corrected by physiotherapy and exercises, but can make it harder for the newborn to breastfeed and turn their head.
- **Webbing or excess skin** (Figure 42.2): this may be folds that can be extended digitally or taut skin areas. It may also be linked to syndromes (e.g. Turner).

Clavicle (collar bone)

The clavicle area should be inspected for shape, distortion and signs of bruising (damaged blood vessels during fracture) (Figure 42.3). Clavicles must also be digitally palpated for presence, size, shape, length, callus (sponge lump) and any crepitus. Crepitus will be felt as a grating sensation where the two ends of the fractured bone meet; movement of the bones may even allow crepitus to be heard. The most common abnormality found is a fracture, but there are other rare abnormalities such as the absence of one or both clavicles (cleidocranial dysostosis) or hypoplasia (congenital pseudoarthrosis).

Fracture (Hashmi et al., 2021)

It is very important that vigilant examination takes place in looking for fractures (Figure 42.4). The clavicle is the most commonly fractured bone at birth. Most are incomplete or 'greenstick' fractures and therefore asymptomatic. Incidence is 4–5 : 1000 births, with 89% identified before discharge – 77% during the physical examination and 23% on incidental X-ray.

A birth history of large baby, caesarean section, ventouse, forceps or extended arms during a breech delivery will increase the incidence of fractures. Be aware that the majority of fractures (77.2%) were seen after spontaneous deliveries, but with 22.8% having a degree of shoulder dystocia, 17.4% occurring after assisted vaginal delivery (forceps or ventouse) and 5.4% following caesarean section. Infants were more commonly male and macrosomic. The affected bone is more commonly on the right side and often the one that was anterior at delivery.

Identification of the fracture was most commonly due to crepitus (57%), swelling and decreased arm movement (20%), swelling only (15%) and incomplete Moro reflex (10%). Inspection may also elicit an irregularity, depression, bruising and puffiness, with signs of pain during the palpation. A callus forms during healing and takes around a week to form, so may be present by the 6-week examination. Brachial nerve injury (Erb's palsy), fracture of the humerus and shoulder dislocation may also be present.

Confirmation is by X-ray. Most fractures heal spontaneously, but awareness will enable monitoring, analgesia and precautions when caring for the newborn. Care includes loose clothing that fully opens and does not require pulling over the head (to reduce the need for movement of the affected arm), no lifting from under the arms and securing the arm by pinning the sleeve to the main body of the garment.

Cleidocranial dysostosis/dysplasia

(Bhattacharya et al., 2023)

This is a rare inherited condition that affects the development of bones along the midline of the skeleton. There can be complete or partial absence of one or both clavicles and small, high scapulae (causing mobile, drooping shoulders). The chest may also have supernumerary ribs, spondylosis and a narrow bell-shaped thorax (with resultant difficulty in breathing). The head may be large with wider fontanelles and suture lines, broad mandible, supernumerary teeth and a high-arched palate. Incomplete bone development can also lead to a wide symphysis, genu valgam (knock knees) and short arms, legs, toes and fingers (e.g. femur, fibula, radius, carpals, tarsals and phalanges).

Congenital pseudoarthrosis (Alsaeed, 2021)

This is a very rare congenital condition in which the clavicle has failed to fuse over ossification points, but it is rarely identified until the child is over 3 years old.

43 Chest

Figure 43.1   Pectus excavatum (pigeon chest) – front view.

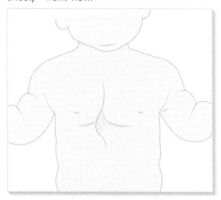

Figure 43.2   Pectus carinatum (barrel chest).

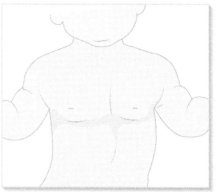

Figure 43.3   AP images of pectus excavatum (top) and pectus carinatum (lower).

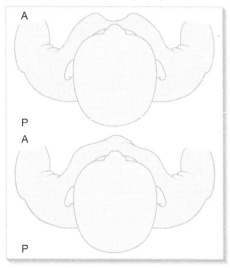

Figure 43.4   True, false and floating ribs.
Source: 4designersart / Adobe Stock.

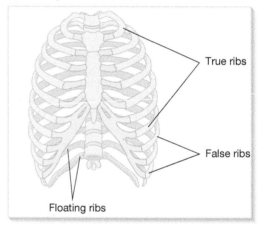

Figure 43.5   Most common line of supernumerary nipples (embryonic milk lines).

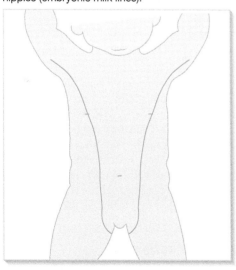

Figure 43.6   Rib abnormalities – bifid, node and notch.

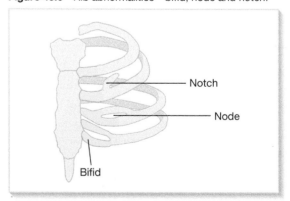

Physical Examination of the Newborn at a Glance, Second Edition. Dr Lyn Dolby and Denise (Dee) Campbell.
© 2025 John Wiley & Sons Ltd. Published 2025 by John Wiley & Sons Ltd.

Chest examination

This chapter considers the inspection and palpation aspects related to the chest. Ideally it will take place when the newborn is quiet, in a warm environment and with the chest and abdomen exposed, with peripheries covered. This will make the examination easier because the chest and abdomen are relaxed. All relevant history and risk factors should be considered in advance.

Chest inspection

Inspection of the chest area considers the colour, appearance and shape of the chest as well as identification of both normal and abnormal features. There should be no abnormal swellings or depressions (see Figures 43.1–43.3). The skin should be pink with no signs of pallor, cyanosis or enlarged, swollen veins. Any evident rashes or birth marks should be assessed fully, but some rashes such as urticaria neonatorum (erythema toxicum) are normal in the 2–5-day-old newborn. Cracking and peeling of the skin are also possible if the newborn was postmature.

The reduced fatty tissue of the newborn and slight intercostal recession may allow some of the ribs to be partially visible against the skin. There are 12 pairs of ribs connected to the vertebra posteriorly. The anterior portions of these ribs are cartilaginous and only the upper 7 pairs are true ribs (reaching the sternum); 8–10 are false ribs (connected to the seventh rib) and 11–12 are floating ribs (not attached to the sternum or other ribs; Figure 43.4). Both sides of the chest should be symmetrical and the chest circumference should appear similar or only slightly larger than the abdomen. These should be measured if there is any uncertainty. In a term infant, 31–33 cm is normal, or approximately 2 cm smaller than the head circumference.

There should be two nipples evident. In the newborn these are small pits in the centre of the areola; nipples evert shortly after birth. These will be one on each side of the chest, aligned roughly mid-clavicle and at a height just below the axilla. As a result of maternal hormones crossing the placenta in utero, both male and female newborns may have swollen nipples, swollen breasts and lumps under the areola in the breast tissue, and there may even be a milky discharge. These conditions are normal and will resolve spontaneously by the 6-week examination. The practitioner should ensure that there is no redness, inflammation, tenderness, pain or any purulent discharge associated with these swellings.

In some newborns the tip of the xiphisternum will be seen protruding slightly mid-chest. This is a small triangular extension of the lower sternum that is still cartilaginous and mobile at birth. It will later gradually ossify, become an extension of the sternum and become less protuberant.

Abnormalities identified on inspection

• **Respiratory distress** (see Chapter 45): Observe for respiratory difficulties indicated by tachypnoea (increased respiratory rate above 60 bpm in a term baby when awake), shallow breaths, chest retraction (sternum or intercostal region), grunting sounds and bluish tone to the skin. If these are present there is likely also to be nasal flare and bluish lips. Oxygen saturation and blood pressure (BP) levels will be required to complete the assessment. In extreme cases paradoxical respiration is seen: the chest wall moves in the opposite direction to normal breathing (moves in on inspiration and out on expiration).

• **Pectus carinatum** (pigeon chest) (Figures 43.2 and 43.3): The sternum is pushed outwards into a general V-shaped protrusion at the centre of the chest. It is usually mild and asymptomatic at birth but increases with age.
• **Pectus excavatum** (funnel chest) (Figures 43.1 and 43.3): The sternum is sunken in the chest causing a visible central depression. This can vary in size but rarely restricts the efficiency of the heart or lungs in a newborn. It may be seen in association with skeletal syndromes (e.g. Marfan syndrome). Restrictions on lung capacity and pressure on the heart may occur later in life, particularly during exercise.
• **Pneumothorax**: An asymmetrical, enlarged anteroposterior diameter is seen. This can occur spontaneously in an otherwise healthy newborn.
• **Poland syndrome**: Under-development of one side of the chest is seen, including ribs, muscle and breast tissue. The syndrome can also affect the upper limb on the affected side.
• **Supernumerary nipples** (Figure 43.5): These are a common minor disorder. Variations occur that include nipples only, areola only, and nipples and areola, and some may include breast tissue (polymastia). They most commonly occur along the embryonic milk lines (Figure 43.5), but can occur anywhere on the chest and down the abdomen, even into the groin.
• **Widely spaced nipples**: This is when nipple spacing is greater than the other percentile measurements for that baby. Nipple spacing ranges from around 7.5 to 9.5 cm apart (3rd to 97th percentile), linked to birth weight and maturity. Wider spacing can be associated with chromosomal abnormality (e.g. Turner syndrome).

Chest palpation

Palpation of the chest should ensure that the skin feels warm. Feel across the ribs and sternum for evidence of masses, crepitus, thrills or of pain in reaction to touch. It is unlikely that the practitioner will be able to identify an increased or decreased number of ribs (sometimes associated with trisomy 21), but a severe malalignment or short ribs/short sternum may become evident through reduced chest circumference combined with palpation. If the xiphisternum is protruding then this should be moveable with gentle pressure to ensure it is not a mass.

Abnormalities identified by palpation

• **Abnormal ribs** (fused, bifid, widened or thin ribs; Figure 43.6) may palpate like a mass on the chest wall, or as reduced or widened intercostal spaces, and are associated with a number of conditions including achondroplasia, osteogenesis imperfecta (also associated with fractures), trisomy 18, rickets and hyperparathyroidism.
• **Emphysema** is trapped subcutaneous air that has escaped from the lungs and may be palpated as crepitus. It may result from overinflation of the lungs (during resuscitation), rib fracture or pneumothorax. Respiratory symptoms of wheezing, tachypnoea and cyanosis will be evident.
• **Fractures** may palpate as crepitus (crackling/popping feeling) when the two ends of bone rub against each other. They may be associated with resuscitation, difficult delivery or osteogenesis imperfecta.
• **Chest masses** are uncommon but when they do occur are more often benign and will have caused rib abnormalities.
• **Thrill** is a vibration that can be palpated through the chest wall, associated with congenital cardiac abnormalities and murmurs.

Cardiovascular assessment

Table 44.1 Key risk factors for congenital heart defects (CHDs).

Risk factor
First-degree relative with a history of CHD (Maternal or sibling increases the risk the most from 5% to 10%)
Foetal trisomy 21 or other diagnosed trisomy (e.g. trisomy 13 or 18)
Cardiac abnormality suspected during antenatal fetal anomaly screening programme (FASP) scan
Other factors associated with CHD such as maternal rubella, diabetes (type 1), epilepsy, systemic lupus erythematosus and drug-related teratogens (e.g. anti-epileptic and psychotic drugs)

Box 44.1 Percentage risk of congenital heart defects for genetic conditions.

- Trisomy 12 (Patau) = 90% risk
- Trisomy 18 (Edwards) = 85% risk
- Trisomy 21 (Down) = 40–50% risk
- Turner syndrome = 35% risk
- Klinefelter syndrome = 15% risk

Table 44.3 Auscultation sites.

Sounds/murmurs arising from	At each point assess for strength, rhythm, volume and any extraneous sounds) Listen with diaphragm of stethoscope in each area and then retrace steps using the bell of the stethoscope
1 Apex (mitral area)	Point of maximum impulse Count heart rate for 1 min and record Left, fifth intercostal space
2 Tricuspid	Lower left sternal border in the fourth intercostal space
3 Pulmonary area	Second intercostal space, left sternal border
4 Aortic area	Second intercostal space, right sternal border Move stethoscope slightly so that respirations can be more clearly heard, count for 1 min and record
5 Area of aortic coarctation	Mid-scapulae Tilt baby gently to insert diaphragm of stethoscope between shoulder blades

Box 44.2 Screen positive findings.

- Tachypnoea at rest
- Episodes of apnoea ≥20 sec or associated with colour change
- Intercostal, subcostal, sternal or supra-sternal recession, nasal flaring
- Central cyanosis
- Visible pulsations over the precordium, heaves, thrills
- Absent or weak femoral pulses
- Presence of cardiac murmurs and/or extra heart sounds

Table 44.2 Key points of cardiovascular examination.

Comprehensive discussion must occur with parent(s) regarding history, developmental processes, parental concerns and what the examination entails		
Observation	General tone	Is the baby floppy?
	Colour (central and peripheral)	Observe colour in daylight. Some babies will exhibit 'acrocyanosis' – a normal phenomenon associated with blue hands and feet after birth
	Size and shape of chest	Should be of normal appearance, not barrel shaped etc.
	Symmetry of chest movement	Movement should be equal on both sides of the baby's chest and there should be no sign of chest recession at the intercostal level (primary) or diaphragm (secondary)
	Respiratory rate	Note rhythm and record rate
	Signs of respiratory distress	No sign of chest recession, nasal flaring or grunting
Palpation	Femoral and brachial pulses	Note strength, rhythm and volume
	Capillary refill time	Depress the nail on the big toe or press gently over the chest – capillary refill time in a neonate should occur within 2 sec
	Position of cardiac apex Presence of heave (strong impulse)	To exclude dextrocardia (heart positioned on the baby's right), tension pneumothorax or diaphragmatic hernia that will be linked to respiratory issues Obvious presence of cardiac impulse may indicate a heart that is working harder than it should
	Presence of thrills	Palpable vibration-like murmur (felt with side edge of hand) similar to cat purring Denotes a grade 1V murmur
	Size of liver	To exclude hepatomegaly, which is associated with congestive cardiac failure
Auscultation	Presence of murmur?	Determine if systolic or diastolic and if loud or quiet

Physical Examination of the Newborn at a Glance, Second Edition. Dr Lyn Dolby and Denise (Dee) Campbell.
© 2025 John Wiley & Sons Ltd. Published 2025 by John Wiley & Sons Ltd.

A

pproximately 1 in 200 babies has a heart anomaly and the comprehensive physical assessment of the neonatal cardiovascular system can assist in the detection of congenital heart defects (CHDs). Overall, the incidence of CHD is approximately 4–10 per 1000 live births, ranging from the non-significant to major and critical anomalies. The critical or major congenital anomalies account for approximately 2–3 per 1000 live births. This latter group constitute the leading cause of morbidity and mortality during and after the neonatal period and is further defined by Public Health England (PHE, 2021a) as:

- **Critical CHD:** includes all potentially life-threatening duct-dependent conditions and those conditions that require procedures within the first 28 days of life.
- **Major serious CHD:** those defects not classified as critical but that require invasive intervention during the first year of life.

Part of the foetal anomaly ultrasound scan encompasses the fetal anomaly screening programme (FASP), which detects a proportion of critical and major cardiac lesions during pregnancy. However, the 'minimum' acceptable FASP standard detection rate for specific cardiac abnormality remains at ≥50%. As the neonatal cardiovascular system is still adapting and changing to extrauterine life, a single examination within the first 72 hours of life may not identify all heart anomalies due to the ongoing developmental processes within the body organs.

Practitioners need to be conversant with the NIPE newborn heart screening: screen positive pathway (PHE, 2021e).

Risk factors

The key risk factors (PHE, 2021a) for CHD are as highlighted in Table 44.1. Also, there is a recognised percentage of risk for CHD in babies born with particular syndromes, which are highlighted in Box 44.1.

Cardiovascular assessment

It is important that the neonatal cardiovascular examination is comprehensive, detailed and that the NIPE practitioner is highly observant during the examination, while taking into account of whether there are any family, antenatal or intrapartum risk factors of relevance.

Ask the parent(s) if there is any history of CHD within the immediate family, as this may not have been noted within the maternal record. The parent(s) should be asked if they have any concerns about their baby's health, such as if the baby ever appears breathless or changes colour when feeding, is not feeding well, is too tired to feed, is quiet or lethargic or has poor muscle tone.

Parents need to be informed that the baby's cardiovascular and respiratory systems are still undergoing changes from intrauterine to extrauterine life. They need to know that as these changes occur it is possible that some murmurs may be heard on auscultation or may not be heard until a certain point of development. If the cardiac auscultation is occurring only a few hours after delivery, the parents need to be prepared that hearing cardiac murmurs on auscultation is more likely. It should be explained that sometimes if the baby is restless, then it may take longer to hear the heart sounds clearly.

Examination process

From the moment the NIPE practitioner first sees the baby until the examination is completed and they walk away, cardiovascular assessment is continuous. This is because throughout the examination, the practitioner should be constantly assessing how the baby is reacting to increased energy and oxygen requirements as they wake, move and interact with the surrounding environment. Table 44.2 highlights the key elements of the examination process, which include observation, palpation and auscultation.

Gaining the skill to palpate very small pulse points takes some practitioners longer to master than others. Bear in mind that neonatal blood pressure is lower and therefore it is easy to occlude a pulse using very little pressure. The ability to palpate the pedal pulses in the baby's foot can prove useful if palpating the femoral pulse is proving difficult, by helping the practitioner to relax and pick up the rhythm of the pulsation.

Link findings relating to the cardiac examination to other elements of the examination process. For example, finding hepatomegaly (enlarged liver) on abdominal palpation may link to other findings associated with congestive cardiac failure. Also, it is the practitioner's responsibility to observe for particular signs that may be indicative of critical or major CHD (see Box 44.1).

When auscultating the chest, make sure that you record the heart rate, which should be in the range of 100–160/minute, and the respiratory rate, which should be in the region of 30–60/minute; both should be listened to for 1 minute. The four main auscultation sites aim for effective cardiac auscultation (Table 44.3) and a fifth site between the shoulder blades (mid-scapulae) assists in hearing murmurs that are associated with coarctation. Use an infant-sized stethoscope, diaphragm first (detects low-pitched sounds), to auscultate sites 1–4, count the heart rate at site 1 and pause at site 4 to listen to the respiratory air entry. Then use the bell (detects high-pitched sounds) to auscultate sites 1–4 in reverse.

Examination findings

- **Screen negative:** No anomalies found during the cardiovascular examination. Baby's next examination will occur in 6–8 weeks with the GP unless the parent(s) are concerned.
- **Screen positive:** Findings include one or more of the signs and symptoms listed in Box 44.2 that could be suggestive of critical or major congenital heart anomalies (PHE, 2021a). Significant murmurs are usually loud, harsh in quality, can be heard over a wide area and are often associated with other abnormal findings. Benign murmurs are typically soft, short, systolic based, localised to the left sternum border and are not associated with other sounds or abnormal findings.

Discuss abnormal findings with a senior paediatrician (neonatologist) or one with expertise in cardiology. The urgency of this consultation will often depend on the clinical condition of the baby, thus any baby where a major or critical condition is suspected must be seen as a matter of urgency. Depending on local Trust policy, initial activity often requires measurement of arterial oxygen saturation (via pulse oximetry) soon after the examination. Public Health England (PHE, 2017) issued an update in relation to a pilot study on the efficacy of pulse oximetry, but since then pulse oximetry has been found to increase the detection of critical congenital heart defects by 96% (Kirk et al., 2022) and its use has been recommended as part of normal postnatal practice (Regan and Monnelly, 2023). However, it is important for all students and staff to be fully conversant with how to apply the equipment used to enable an accurate assessment.

Communication with parents

Cardiac anomalies can create life-changing conditions for both the baby and the parent(s). The impact on a parent as a result of a referral for suspected CHD can be profound and referral needs to be expedited smoothly and efficiently, with adequate explanation regarding the reason behind the referral, what will happen and when. Most Trust sites have protocols in place for staff to follow and therefore they should be conversant with the actions that need to be taken and why.

All parents must be given comprehensive information relating to the signs and symptoms of ill health that they need to be aware of (see Chapter 6), whether their baby is considered to be at risk or not, due to the developmental changes continuing to occur over the next few weeks. Therefore, it is paramount to make sure that parents know when to call for an ambulance and the contact numbers for enquiries of a less serious nature.

45 Respiratory assessment and hypoxia

Figure 45.1 Subcostal recession during inspiration.

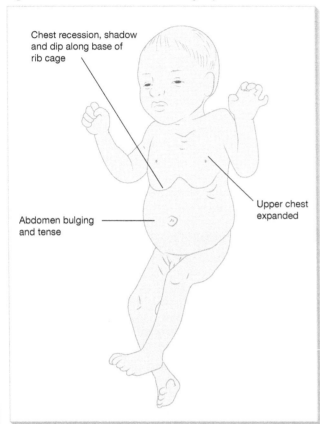

Chest recession, shadow and dip along base of rib cage

Upper chest expanded

Abdomen bulging and tense

Figure 45.2 Intercostal recession during inspiration extending to the sternum.

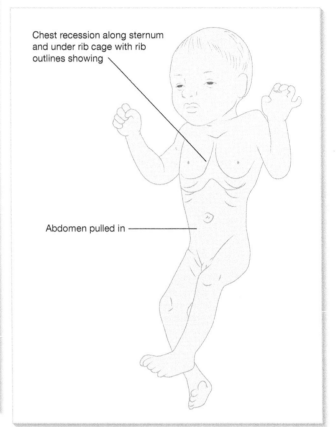

Chest recession along sternum and under rib cage with rib outlines showing

Abdomen pulled in

Figure 45.3 Sites of possible congenital airway stenosis from larynx to bronchi.

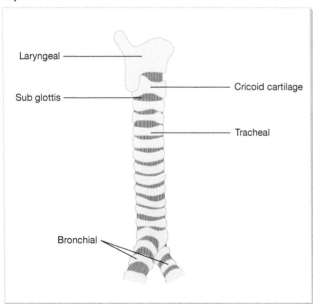

Laryngeal

Sub glottis

Cricoid cartilage

Tracheal

Bronchial

Figure 45.4 Normal nasal passages showing choanal atresia.

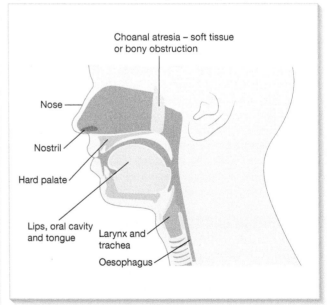

Choanal atresia – soft tissue or bony obstruction

Nose

Nostril

Hard palate

Lips, oral cavity and tongue

Larynx and trachea

Oesophagus

Physical Examination of the Newborn at a Glance, Second Edition. Dr Lyn Dolby and Denise (Dee) Campbell.
© 2025 John Wiley & Sons Ltd. Published 2025 by John Wiley & Sons Ltd.

Respiratory assessment

Respiratory assessment includes observation of chest movement, auscultation of breath sounds and evaluation of other signs of respiratory problems. The infant needs to be undressed in a warm environment with peripheries covered to prevent respiratory changes because they are cold. As the ribs are still partially cartilaginous and weak, breathing is abdominal and diaphragmatic. As a result, it is the abdomen that can be seen expanding during respiration and the lower thorax may pull in slightly. Nose breathing occurs when babies are quiet, but they breathe through the mouth when crying. A normal feeding pattern is reassuring, as respiratory problems are exacerbated during feeding. Respiratory issues are rarely concealed so should become evident on examination, but it should be appreciated that they may be a symptom of problems outside of the respiratory tract (e.g. cardiac anomalies).

Inspection

Inspection should confirm relaxed, symmetrical movement at 40–60 respirations timed over a full minute when awake and 30–40 when asleep. The newborn should have the same normal skin colour over the whole body. Peripheral cyanosis (purple-blue discolouration to lighter skins, but may be grey or white to darker skins) of the hands, feet and nail beds may occur, but should not extend centrally, nor to the lips, tongue or mucous membranes. Pallor precedes cyanosis so is also significant. Breathing should not appear to require effort, so there should be no nasal flare and any chest recession on inspiration should be very mild and intercostal. It should not extend to the sternum nor should there be deep intercostal or subcostal recession (Figures 45.1 and 45.2). Breathing is generally regular; however, a short episode of erratic breathing and even a 10-second apnoea can be normal. If any irregularity occurs, extend the time observing until reassured; include pulse oximetry and consider chest X-ray.

Auscultation

Auscultation of breath sounds requires a quiet environment and should be via both the bell and the diaphragm of the stethoscope. At the initial examination, auscultation routinely occurs subclavicle on both sides of the anterior upper chest. By the 6-week examination, when the chest is larger, routine auscultation occurs in the upper, mid and lower chest cavity on both sides and both anteriorly and posteriorly. Auscultation checks that air entry, inspiration and expiration are all symmetrical and that no abnormal sounds are heard. Sounds are coarser and higher pitched nearer the midline, becoming softer and lower pitched further from the sternum. Secretions, foreign bodies or water will make breath sounds harder to hear.

Abnormal breath sounds

There are a number of abnormal breath sounds that can be examined for, but be aware that breath sounds can be normal even in the presence of conditions as severe as pneumonia. Additionally, while abnormality may begin with increased respirations, exhaustion will progress this to slowed respiration and eventual periods of apnoea of 20 seconds or more. Consider the full picture: breath sounds, respiratory rate (and depth), chest recession and any changes during wakeful periods and feeding. If there is any concern, then pulse oximetry is indicated and X-ray may be required.

- **Apnoea**: absence of breathing. Occasional and temporary apnoea (≤10 seconds) can be normal, but may also result from maternal drug use, infection, choanal atresia (Figure 45.4), neurological disease or respiratory distress syndrome.

- **Bradypnoea**: slowed respirations, which may also be shallow as a result of traumatic birth, hypoxia, anoxia or maternal drugs.
- **Crepitations (crackles or rales)**: crackling, clicking or rattling sounds caused by increased lung fluid, e.g. chest infection, pneumonia.
- **Grunting**: expiration through a partially closed glottis. Relatively common and typically resolves spontaneously within two hours, but may also be associated with infection, hypoglycaemia, hernia and respiratory or cardiac disease.
- **Paradoxical respiration**: the chest wall moves in the opposite direction to normal (in on inspiration and out on expiration), e.g. with severe respiratory distress syndrome.
- **Respiratory distress syndrome**: a breathing disorder that is more common with prematurity. Symptoms include tachypnoea, shallow breaths, chest retraction (sternum or intercostal region), grunting sounds, bluish tone to light-coloured skin, white discolouration to dark-coloured skin, nasal flare and bluish lips with paradoxical respiration if severe.
- **Rhonchi**: low-pitched wheeze, like a snoring sound.
- **See-saw respirations**: extreme chest compression and abdominal bulging on inspiration, with extreme abdominal compression on expiration (e.g. during obstructed airway; Figure 45.3).
- **Stridor**: a harsh vibratory or whistling sound on expiration, e.g. during upper-airway obstruction (Figure 45.3).
- **Tachypnoea**: rapid breathing. May be normal before 24 hours (because of retained lung fluid) and resolve spontaneously; otherwise indicates infection, hernia or heart, lung or metabolic disease.
- **Unequal air entry**: may be caused by heart failure, infection, pneumothorax or upper-airway obstruction (Figure 45.3 and 45.4).
- **Wheeze**: high- or low-pitched whistling sound on expiration caused by inflammation or narrowing of large airways (Figure 45.3 and 45.4).

Hypoxia

This is a condition in which oxygen levels to the brain are reduced. More commonly associated with labour, it can also occur postnatally as an acute or slowly progressing condition when abnormalities of the respiratory, cardiovascular, neurological or metabolic systems occur. Early detection and minimising of damage are essential, as the damage cannot be repaired.

Choanal atresia

This is the most common nasal airway obstruction and may be unilateral or bilateral (Figure 45.4). Newborns are normally nose breathers when quiet and mouth breathers when crying. If the condition is bilateral, early cyanosis and apnoea are apparent and nose breathing is not possible. In unilateral cases, obstructing the nostrils in turn will help detect which side is affected, because obstructing the unaffected side will immediately increase symptoms. Immediate referral is required to enable insertion of an oropharyngeal airway and full investigation of the obstruction.

Pulse oximetry

Pulse oximetry is a screening tool for the measurement of oxygen levels in blood using sensors placed on the fingers and toes. An air-breathing newborn aged 2 hours or more should have a minimum 95% oxygen saturation level. Paediatricians are increasingly introducing pulse oximetry as a screening tool. This is despite the UK NSC study considering the feasibility, advantages and disadvantages of using it routinely concluding that the high false-positive reporting rate should delay its routine introduction (PHE, 2017).

46 Upper limbs and hands

Figure 46.1 Normal palmar creases.

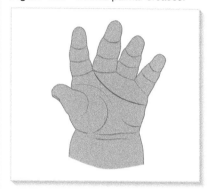

Figure 46.2 Bones of the upper limb and hand.

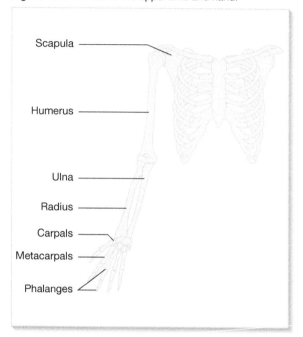

Scapula

Humerus

Ulna

Radius

Carpals

Metacarpals

Phalanges

Figure 46.3 Erb's palsy.

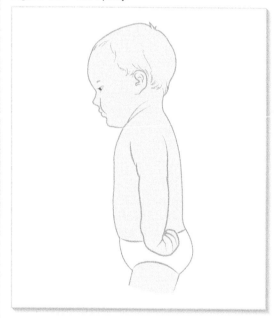

Figure 46.4 Oligodactyly (missing fingers).

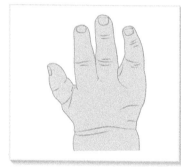

Figure 46.5 Polydactyly (additional fingers).

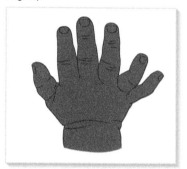

Figure 46.6 Single simian crease.

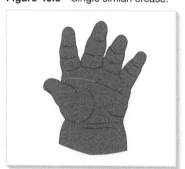

Figure 46.7 Sydney line.

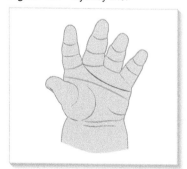

Figure 46.8 Syndactyly (joined fingers).

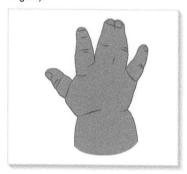

Physical Examination of the Newborn at a Glance, Second Edition. Dr Lyn Dolby and Denise (Dee) Campbell.
© 2025 John Wiley & Sons Ltd. Published 2025 by John Wiley & Sons Ltd.

This chapter includes examination of the shoulders, arms and hands (Figures 46.1 and 46.2). Abnormalities of the upper limbs and hands are associated with a range of causes, including genetic disorders and syndromes (e.g. achondroplasia and Marfan syndrome), hypocalcaemia (e.g. hypoparathyroidism) and amniotic bands. Assessment is of bones, joints, muscles and the skin, as well as checking for symmetry of shape and range of movement across the two arms.

Conditions affecting the upper limbs may also affect the lower limbs. The best known of these is perhaps the thalidomide birth defects from the late 1950s. A sedative, useful in reducing morning sickness, was taken by 12,000 pregnant women worldwide. For almost half of these the result was miscarriage or stillbirth. Surviving babies experienced multiple upper- and lower-limb deformities. Nowadays the most common causes of upper- and lower-limb abnormalities are as follows:

- **Achondroplasia (dwarfism)/Kniest dysplasia (disproportionate dwarfism)**: genetic conditions with the production of calcium and collagen reduced, affecting all bone and joint development. Upper limbs will have bowed bones, enlarged joints and short, fat fingers.
- **Radial or ulnar longitudinal deficiency**: a condition that varies in the extent of abnormality. There is poor development and deformities of the upper limbs and particularly the radius and the hands. In severe cases, the lower arms and joints appear significantly curved as a result of short radius, normal ulna and resultant asymmetrical growth.

Shoulder abnormalities

When examining the shoulder, the most common injuries to be looked for may be identified by the reduced mobility of the affected arm, absence of reflexes and a birth associated with possible trauma.

- **Brachial plexus injury**: damage to the brachial plexus nerve group through stretching of the nerve roots, which leads to partial or full muscle weakness down the arm and possibly a paralysed arm. Moro and grasp reflexes will be poor or absent and Erb's or Klumpke's palsy may be evident. Spontaneous recovery is common, supported by physiotherapy by the parent(s), but may take 6 months. If no recovery is evident by this time then surgery may be required and the prognosis for full recovery becomes poor.
- **Erb's palsy** (Figure 46.3): resulting from a high brachial plexus injury, recognised by the 'waiter's tip' positioning. This is when the limp arm rotates inward slightly, with loss of flexion at the elbow, and the hand flexes at the wrist to face backwards and upwards.
- **Klumpke's palsy**: resulting from a low brachial plexus injury and affecting the forearm and hand, with muscle damage causing a 'clawed hand' shape.
- **Dislocated shoulders**: rare, resulting from direct trauma at birth, brachial plexus injury or as a congenital defect. Dislocations are recognised by internal rotation of the arm, flexion of the wrist and a normal grasp but absent Moro reflex. Movement is limited and asymmetrical, with sensation apparent through evidence of pain. The affected shoulder may appear flatter than the unaffected side.

Arms

Examination of the arms inspects for fractures (humerus, radius or ulna), dislocated elbow and abnormalities, with awareness that the elbow will not completely straighten due to a mild flexion contracture (Figure 46.2).

- **Amniotic constriction band**: fibrous bands from the amnion wrap around the developing fetus inhibiting growth, from slight indentations to complete prevention of limb formation.
- **Dislocated elbow**: when the radius and/or the ulna have been pulled out of line from the humerus. It is a very rare birth injury recognised by immobility, pain and malalignment.
- **Fractures**: a fractured humerus is the second most common fracture for a newborn after the clavicle. Fractures of the radius or ulna are rare. Indicators are traumatic delivery, caesarean section, restricted movement and pain. It is rarely possible to detect a fracture (unless there is significant malalignment) until a callus forms 7–10 days later.
- **Limb-reduction defects**: affect either upper or lower limbs and occasionally upper and lower at the same time.
- **Tumours**: growths that may be deeper within the arm or on the skin (e.g. haemangioma).

Hands and fingers

When examining the hands, each finger and the thumb must be opened fully and inspected along to the nails. The palm, back and sides of the hand must all be checked. Nails can be soft, but should be smooth and extend to the finger tips. The normal hand position is in a fist with the thumb tucked in, but a persistent fist may be a sign of nerve damage. Techniques to encourage the hand to open include stroking either the back of the hand or the ulnar side. Abnormalities may be individual or part of a syndrome and include the following:

- **Absent or deformed nails**: may be nail-patella syndrome.
- **Arachnodactyly (spider legs)**: long, thin fingers. Associated with connective tissue disorders (e.g. Marfan syndrome).
- **Brachydactyly**: short fingers.
- **Camptodactyly**: abnormally bent fingers; fixed flexion.
- **Clinodactyly**: a curving finger; may cause overlapping.
- **Kniest dysplasia**: long, knobbly fingers and no fist shape.
- **Macrodactyly**: one or more enlarged fingers.
- **Oligodactyly**: one or more absent digits (Figure 46.4).
- **Overlapping**: flexed fingers rarely overlap. If the index finger overlaps this can be associated with trisomy 18.
- **Polydactyly**: one or more extra digits (Figure 46.5).
- **Short, fat digits**: seen in achondroplasia and hypoparathyroidism.
- **Simian crease** (Figure 46.6): single palmar crease, commonly associated with trisomy 21 (short finger, incurved little finger and low-set thumb also likely). Occurs with many other genetic conditions and in a small number of unaffected newborns.
- **Sydney line** (Figure 46.7): like the simian crease this is associated with trisomy 21 and also congenital rubella.
- **Symbrachdactyly**: short fingers, plus webbing.
- **Syndactyly** (Figure 46.8): fused fingers; may be at skin level or include bone.
- **Trident hand deformity**: low attachment of thumb, third and fourth fingers project laterally, associated with achondroplasia.
- **Webbing**: may be reduced (limiting movement) or increased (either extending up the length of the finger or as excessive folds).

47 Abdomen

Figure 47.1 Gastroschisis.
Source: Reproduced with permission from Lissauer et al. (2020) / John Wiley & Sons.

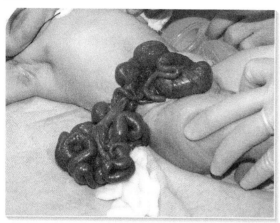

Figure 47.2 Types of oesophageal atresia.
Source: Reproduced with permission from Lissauer et al. (2020) / John Wiley & Sons.

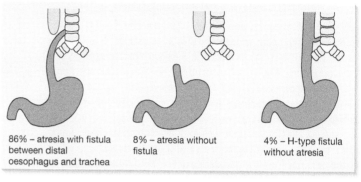

86% – atresia with fistula between distal oesophagus and trachea

8% – atresia without fistula

4% – H-type fistula without atresia

Figure 47.3 Frothy oral secretions linked to oesophageal atresia.
Source: Reproduced with permission from Lissauer et al. (2020) / John Wiley & Sons.

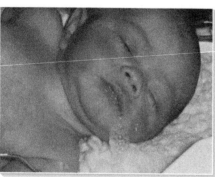

Figure 47.4 Omphalocele.
Source: Reproduced with permission from Lissauer et al. (2020) / John Wiley & Sons.

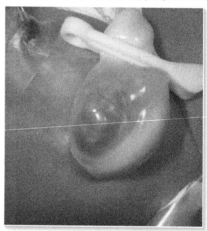

Figure 47.6 Abdominal masses and their causes.
Source: Reproduced with permission from Lissauer et al. (2020) / John Wiley & Sons.

Figure 47.5 Quadrants of abdomen and aspects palpable.

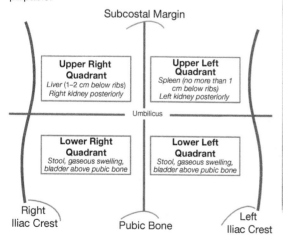

Subcostal Margin

Upper Right Quadrant	Upper Left Quadrant
Liver (1–2 cm below ribs) Right kidney posteriorly	Spleen (no more than 1 cm below ribs) Left kidney posteriorly

Umbilicus

Lower Right Quadrant	Lower Left Quadrant
Stool, gaseous swelling, bladder above pubic bone	Stool, gaseous swelling, bladder above pubic bone

Right Iliac Crest

Pubic Bone

Left Iliac Crest

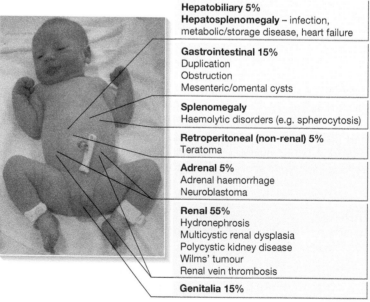

Hepatobiliary 5%
Hepatosplenomegaly – infection, metabolic/storage disease, heart failure

Gastrointestinal 15%
Duplication
Obstruction
Mesenteric/omental cysts

Splenomegaly
Haemolytic disorders (e.g. spherocytosis)

Retroperitoneal (non-renal) 5%
Teratoma

Adrenal 5%
Adrenal haemorrhage
Neuroblastoma

Renal 55%
Hydronephrosis
Multicystic renal dysplasia
Polycystic kidney disease
Wilms' tumour
Renal vein thrombosis

Genitalia 15%

Physical Examination of the Newborn at a Glance, Second Edition. Dr Lyn Dolby and Denise (Dee) Campbell.
© 2025 John Wiley & Sons Ltd. Published 2025 by John Wiley & Sons Ltd.

Abdominal examination

This chapter considers the inspection and palpation aspects related to the abdomen. Ideally, the examination should take place when the newborn is quiet, in a warm environment, with the chest and abdomen exposed and peripheries covered. This will make the examination easier since the chest and abdomen are relaxed. All relevant history and risk factors should be considered in advance, paying particular attention to ultrasound results regarding any organ abnormalities or polyhydramnios detected (associated with increased risk of oesophageal and duodenal atresia). It will be important to ask about feeding, stools and micturition patterns, as well as inspecting any evidence of vomiting.

Abdominal inspection

Inspection of the abdomen examines for colour, size, shape, symmetry, movement and evidence of any abnormality. The skin should be skin color and the abdomen should appear soft and symmetrically rounded, without swelling or depression. The abdominal muscles and skin should appear well toned. Some flattening or distension is possible linked to time of last feed, but the abdominal circumference typically remains between 31 and 34 cm for a term infant. As the newborn is a diaphragmatic breather, it is normal for the abdomen to move more than the chest during respirations.

The umbilical area should be dry, with no offensive odour or discharge. If the examination is on the day of birth, then identify the two arteries and one vein. If a single artery is seen or identified at birth, ensure urine has been passed and antenatal ultrasound was normal. Any green discolouration may indicate meconium passed in utero, so check the intrapartum history. A clean, healthy, umbilical stump is dry by the second postnatal day and has separated by 10–12 days.

Abnormalities seen on inspection

Many abnormalities are so obvious they are identified at or shortly after birth such as gastroschisis (Figure 47.1), bladder exstrophy, ascites, hydrops fetalis, necrotising enterocolitis, malrotation and volvulus. Other abnormalities become obvious once feeding commences or symptoms worsen:
- **Abnormal colour**: duskiness of a light-coloured skin or whitening of a dark-coloured skin indicates poor circulation or bowel necrosis; redness indicates inflamed bowel.
- **Diaphragmatic hernia**: weakness of diaphragm muscles causes scaphoid (sunken) abdomen; allows organs to push into chest cavity.
- **Diastasis recti**: separated rectus abdominus muscle allows protrusion down the central line of the abdomen particularly during crying; corrects naturally.
- **Duodenal atresia**: closed part of the duodenum; upper abdominal distension; vomiting (even long after feeds); urination and bowel movements stop after the first few.
- **Epigastric hernia**: small, firm, palpable, nodule between the xiphoid process and the umbilicus; fat protruding through muscle weakness.
- **Hirschsprung's disease**: absence of nerve cells regulating colon; affects short or long portion; obstruction, distension, failure to pass meconium and green or brown vomit.
- **Meconium ileus**: distended abdomen and meconium impaction. Most are associated with cystic fibrosis.

- **Oesophageal atresia/tracheoesophageal fistula** (Figures 47.2 and 47.3): oesophageal obstruction, often with missing portion; commonly with fistula to trachea; distension; frothy oral secretion.
- **Omphalitis**: redness and inflammation of the umbilicus; can track back into the abdomen if not managed early.
- **Omphalocele** (Figure 47.4): herniation of abdominal contents into the umbilical cord, surrounded by clear sac.
- **Organomegaly**: enlarged organs causing abdominal distension.
- **Prune (wrinkled) belly**: reduced musculature of abdomen.
- **Supernumerary nipples**: may occur on the abdomen.
- **Umbilical granuloma**: excessive granulation causes a red, fleshy swelling of the umbilicus; most resolve spontaneously.
- **Umbilical hernia**: weak musculature around the umbilicus; may also allow abdominal contents to protrude.
- **Urachal cyst, sinus or fistula**: clear fluid or urine draining from an opening onto the abdomen between the bladder and the umbilicus.

Palpation of the abdomen

Palpation can confirm concerns following inspection, but also checks for masses, organomegaly, tense or relaxed musculature, retained urine or stool, signs of pain or another abnormality. Palpate all four quadrants and centrally (Figure 47.5). Begin gently, to allow the newborn to become tolerant and not distressed, then deeper palpation will be possible. It is normal to feel some gaseous distension, stool and bladder in the lower quadrants. Upper organs, not entirely covered by the rib cage, can be felt in the upper quadrants.

To palpate, stand to the side of the newborn. Apply the flat, palmar surface of the four fingers and progress in a rolling movement upwards, from the iliac crest to the subcostal margin. Begin in the lower right quadrant. Depress 1–2 cm only and do not lift the fingers completely off, because this will risk missing an area. The liver will be identified in the upper quadrant, 1–2 cm below the ribs; it has a smooth firm edge and should not feel nodular or hard. Next palpate the left side; it is rare to feel the spleen but, if felt, it must not be more than 1 cm below the ribs. To ensure it is the spleen, feel for a notch in its shape and check it moves with respirations. To feel for the kidneys, place a hand under the infant's back between the false ribs and waist to ballot the kidney forward. Press down on the abdomen with the second hand, lateral to the umbilicus, at a 45° angle. Each kidney is about 4–5 cm long and feels like a smooth, firm flattened plum. The right kidney is lower and easier to feel. Lastly, feel for a bladder. Begin at the umbilicus and palpate downwards, feeling for a fullness rising out of the pelvis. It may be felt 1–4 cm above the symphysis pubis but should not be a permanent feature. Typically, urination occurs within the first 12 hours of birth and occurs five times over the first 48 hours of life.

Abnormalities detected on palpation

- **Hepatomegaly**: enlarged liver.
- **Hydronephrosis**: enlarged kidney resulting from fluid. May resolve spontaneously if urine and not a result of malformation, tumours, polycystic kidneys or infection.
- **Masses** (Figure 47.6): any nodules felt on any organ.
- **Pyloric stenosis**: a firm, oval-shaped mass in the upper mid-abdomen; not present at birth but may be felt at 6 weeks.
- **Splenomegaly** (Figure 47.6): enlarged spleen.
- **Tenderness**: distress and drawing up of knees during palpation may be a pain reaction.

48 Back, spine, buttocks and anus

Figure 48.1   Normal curvature of spine. (a) Adult. (b) Newborn.
Source: Injurymap / CC BY 2.0.

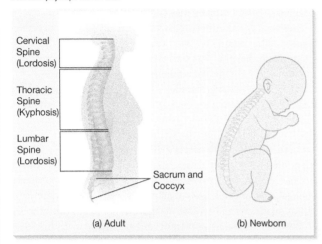

Figure 48.2   Image of a newborn caudal appendage (tail).

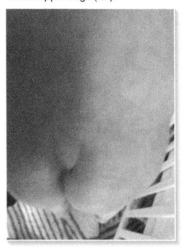

Figure 48.3   Occipital encephalocele.
Source: Reproduced with permission from Lissauer et al. (2020) / John Wiley & Sons.

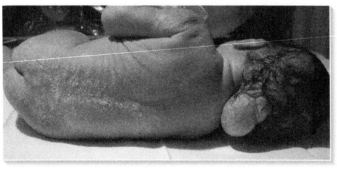

Figure 48.4   Spina bifida occulta, a defect in vertebrae – without spinal cord damage or prolapse of meninges.
Source: Lissauer et al. (2020) / John Wiley & Sons.

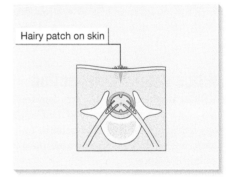

Figure 48.5   Meningocele, a defect in vertebrae with prolapse of meninges – without spinal cord damage. CSF, cerebro-spinal fluid.
Source: Lissauer et al. (2020) / John Wiley & Sons.

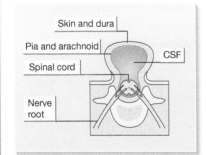

Figure 48.6   Myelomeningocele, a defect in vertebrae and skin – with prolapse of meninges and spinal cord.
Source: Lissauer et al. (2020) / John Wiley & Sons.

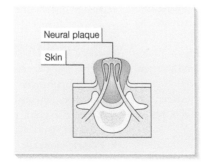

Figure 48.7   Myelomeningocele.
Source: Lissauer et al. (2020) / John Wiley & Sons.

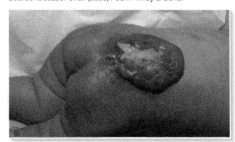

The examination begins with awareness of the history for any risk factors, paying particular attention to anomaly screening, for instance nuchal space, banana or lemon sign, sibling history, anticonvulsant therapy, alpha-fetoprotein (AFP). Reassuring factors include antenatal folic acid therapy and normal head and neck. Antenatal management makes it unlikely that major abnormalities will remain undetected. However, not all women accept screening and false negatives can occur (e.g. skin-covered spinal lesions will not raise AFP levels). Signs that are not detected antenatally will be the less obvious ones, making care during this examination even more important.

Working in a light, warm environment, lie the newborn prone over your hand and lower forearm. Inspect for changes in normal skin colour, hairy patches (other than lanugo), deformity, dimples (of any depth), masses and evidence of a normally situated patent anus. Visualising the passage of stool will be a reassuring feature. Palpation covers the whole back and full length of the spine, ensuring normal curvature and that all spinal processes are felt.

Back

The back is examined for any abnormalities of the skin, curvature and scapulae. The back of a newborn baby does not have changes in curvature Figure 48.1. The prone position, lying over the forearm, should enable confirmation that the back is convex (Figure 48.1). The skin should have no birth marks or evidence of masses. It is covered in inconspicuous fine hairs but may also have noticeable downy unpigmented hair (lanugo) for a few weeks. Dark hairs may be seen on Asian babies – wider cuticles make the hair more noticeable. Excessive hair may relate to hormone imbalance and requires investigation. The scapulae (shoulder bones) should be roughly triangular in shape, with a flat surface. The upper border is roughly horizontal, below clavicle height and with normal shoulder movement.

- **Congenital dermal melanocytosis (Hyperpigmented macule)**: can occur in single or multiple patches. Document their presence to ensure they are not mistaken for bruising and abuse, occasionally they are associated with underlying concerns (see chapter 37).
- **Sprengel's deformity**: small, winged or raised scapulae with the lower point protruding; typically unilateral, making the scapulae asymmetrical. A raised effect may make the neck appear webbed and limits movement. Check for scoliosis and Klippel-Feil syndrome.

Spine

Examine from the base of the skull to the coccyx, looking and feeling for changes to the skin colour or texture, tufts of hair, soft or cystic masses, dimples, cysts or sinus tracts. The most common congenital spinal deformities are associated with abnormal or incomplete development or postural deformities.

Spinal curvature

Congenital spinal curvature may be secondary to in utero positioning or associated with abnormally fused vertebrae. Sitting the infant resting over one hand will sometimes make kyphosis or lordosis more apparent and holding under the arms and raising the infant may make a scoliosis more obvious. Early detection allows corrective management before growth exaggerates the problem. The three main curvatures are:
- **Kyphosis**: exaggerated curvature of thoracic and sacral regions.
- **Lordosis**: exaggerated curvature of lower, lumbar region.
- **Scoliosis**: sideways curvature of the spine to left or right.

Caudal appendage (tail) (Rueda et al., 2022) (Figure 48.2)

Caudal appendages are more commonly found with male newborns and may be identified at any point between the lumbar and peri-anal region. They can be up to 20 cm long. True or vestigial tails contain connective tissue, fat, muscle, nerves and blood vessels but no vertebrae or bone. Pseudo tails also contain bone and cartilage and can be associated with numerous disorders, such as incomplete fusion of the spine, teratoma, lipoma, spinal cord anomalies, tethered cord syndrome and spina bifida occulta (SBO). Management includes assessment for underlying problems and may require surgical removal of the appendage if its position will affect physical or psychological health.

Spinal neural tube disorders

SBO and spina bifida cystica (SBC) are the two main disorders, but an encephalocele (Figure 48.3) may occur at the top of the spine where the skull and spine meet. Concerns arise if a lump, dimple, hairy patch or naevus is seen over the midline and these require further investigation.
- **SBO** (Figure 48.4): incomplete closure of one or more vertebrae; often asymptomatic as cord is intact; risks increase depending on the size of the defect and number of vertebrae affected. Those that are more extensive are associated with a dimple, sinus, hair tuft, naevus, or fatty swelling (lipomyelomeningocele).
- **SBC**: incomplete closure of one or more vertebrae with varying degrees of protrusion of the cord and meninges. Most are lumbosacral.
  - **Meningocele** (Figure 48.5): protrusion of meninges with normal underlying spinal cord; can be dura or skin covered.
  - **Myelomeningocele** (Figures 48.6 and 48.7): protrusion of meninges and spinal cord; most in a sealed sac of cerebro-spinal fluid (CSF); flat or bulging. Check for CSF leakage, hydrocephalus, orthopaedic or neurological abnormalities (lower-limb paralysis).
  - **Myeloschisis**: a myelomeningocele where a mass of nerve tissue has flattened along the skin surface.
- **Spinal or dermal dimple**: commonly an innocent sacro-coccygeal dimple, particularly if it lies over the coccyx. It could also indicate an underlying spinal abnormality – SBO or a tethered spinal cord. A tethered cord can be stretched and damaged as the infant grows.
- **Spinal or dermal sinus**: a tract down from the skin; may reach the spinal cord but most end in a cyst or tumour. Can occur anywhere but most are lumbar. Observe for leaking CSF. Do not probe as this may introduce infection or cause further damage. May be associated with a tethered cord.

Buttocks

The most common abnormalities seen are congenital dermal melanocytosis and sacral dimples, but other forms of naevus are possible. A pilonidal dimple is one based above the buttock cleft. Sacral dimples are mostly shallow enough for the base to be seen and are innocent. If it is not possible to see the base then investigate for possible sinus or fistula.

Anus

Examine for position, patency and to ensure there are no associated fistulae. Patency can only be confirmed by witnessing the passage of stool. Evidence of stool in the nappy is reassuring, but not confirmation that it was passed from the anus. Examine dimples to ensure they do not leak stool – a patent anus does not prohibit leakage of stool from a secondary site. Elicit the anal wink reflex (puckering contraction during gentle stimuli) to confirm normal sensory and motor responses and ensure the stool type, quantity and frequency are all normal.

49 Developmental dysplasia of the hips

Table 49.1 Investigate, observe and manipulate.

Investigate			
Prior to examination: Review the family, antenatal, intrapartum and immediate postnatal history for risk factors Discuss rationale for assessing for developmental dysplasia of the hips (DDH) with parent(s) and gain agreement for the two manoeuvres to be performed			

Observe	Screen positive findings are in red		
Normal leg movement when nappy is removed	Does the baby kick and knees abduct naturally? Pay particular attention if one leg is habitually held in an unnatural position		
Symmetry of leg length	The practitioner needs to stand at the baby's feet, ensuring that the baby lies straight	Difference in leg length	
Level of knees when hips and knees are both flexed	Galeazzi or Allis sign – do not just look down at the knees, lower yourself so that you are looking at them on the same level	Knees at different levels when hips and knees are bilaterally flexed	

Manipulate			
Ortolani	Screens for a dislocated hip	Restricted unilateral limitation of hip abduction with a difference of 20° or more between hips. Gross bilateral limitation of hip abduction (loss of 30° abduction or more) Palpable 'clunk' or 'jerk' is felt A non-smooth rotation of the joint when returning to the neutral position (Figure 44.1(a) may indicate a structural issue and requires referral to a senior paediatrician	
Barlow	Screens for a dislocatable hip	Palpable 'clunk' or 'jerk' is felt	

Notes:
Ortolani is a normal movement for a neonate, but some babies have a natural stricture behind the knee and therefore the hip may not abduct to 90°. Any baby where the hip cannot be abducted to at least 70° should be referred.
Barlow is not a natural movement for a baby, neither is it a manoeuvre that actively seeks to dislocate the hip, but correct positioning of the femur/femoral head during the manoeuvre allows detection of instability and if DDH is present will demonstrate subluxation or dislocation.

Table 49.2   Ortolani and Barlow manoeuvres.

Prior to examination: The baby should be lying on a firm, flat surface, straight, relaxed and free from the nappy or surrounding clothing/bedding. The practitioner should stand at the end of the cot

For both Ortolani and Barlow manoeuvres
Both legs should be gently flexed to a right angle – the legs should not be over- or under-flexed. This is the neutral position from which both manoeuvres commence and finish (Figure 49.1a). In neonates each hip should be examined separately, as this increases effectivity.

Ortolani (Figure 49.1b) *Side being tested*	
	Side not being tested
Place middle finger on the greater trochanter (outer bony prominence near the neck of the femur) with the thumb round the distal, medial femur In a male baby, take care not to catch the scrotal sac	The hand on this side of the baby is used to stabilise the **pelvis,** preventing the baby from rolling sideways as the manoeuvre is performed (which would reduce the ability to assess the full extent of abduction on the side being tested)
Middle finger should apply a slight upward pressure to the greater trochanter as the practitioner's hand rotates the leg/hip outwards until the back of the hand connects with the mattress. The leg should then be returned, in a controlled movement, to its original position, feeling for smoothness of rotation	The hand is applied to the baby in a similar fashion as on the side being tested, but the fingers are slipped under the buttock to hold the pelvis and prevent movement If the baby is fidgety or wishes to kick, the fingers can be placed under the buttocks with the thumb placed firmly, but gently, on the symphysis pubis
A **positive sign** is indicated by a palpable 'clunk', jerk or grating as the hip is abducted and returned to the neutral position	Practitioners who are learning can inadvertently exert more pressure on the symphysis pubis than a more experienced practitioner, thus the former handhold is preferential at first
Barlow (Figure 49.1c) *Side being tested*	
	Side not being tested
The soft tissue between thumb and forefinger of the hand needs to be placed slightly higher than in the starting position for Ortolani. Adduct the knee to the midline and apply pressure downwards and backwards through the axis of the femur. The adducted angle of the femur **must** be maintained until the pressure is released and the leg returned to the neutral position. The femoral head may jerk or a palpable clunk may be felt if it dislocates from the acetabulum – **a positive sign**	Stabilisation of the pelvis is not so important in preventing the pelvis rolling, but rather it holds the pelvis steady, allowing the examining hand to feel the movement of the hip being tested However, the knee/leg on the side not being tested should be allowed to **abduct** slightly in order to give room for the other leg to be adducted. This helps to initiate an effective adduction and to maintain the angle during the manoeuvre

The Barlow manoeuvre is not used to make the hip dislocate but to place it in a position where it might do so if unstable.
The femoral head may be felt to move too easily to the brim of the acetabulum (demonstrating laxity/subluxation), which is often due to the impact of maternal hormones on the neonate during the first 10 days of life.

Figure 49.1   (a) Neutral position; (b) Ortolani manoeuvre; and (c) Barlow manoeuvre.
Source: Lissauer et al. (2020) / John Wiley & Sons.

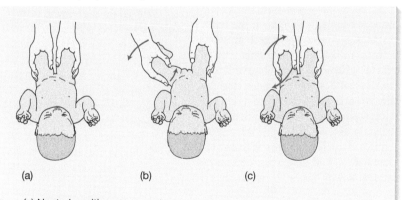

(a)   (b)   (c)

(a) Neutral position
(b) Test for dislocatable hip. The hip is held flexed and adducted to the midline. The femoral head is pushed downwards.
   If dislocatable, the femoral head will be pushed posteriorly out of the acetabulum
(c) Test for dislocated hip. Abduct hip with upward leverage of femur.
   A dislocated hip will return with a palpable **clunk** into the acetabulum

DDH develops when abnormal development occurs between the femoral head and the acetabulum of the pelvis. More specifically, DDH encompasses a spectrum of conditions ranging from minor acetabular dysplasia and laxity to irreducible dislocation of the femoral head. Therefore, assessing hip stability is a primary focus of the NIPE in order that the dislocated or dislocatable hip(s) is identified early, and that an ultrasound scan (USS) is conducted in a timely manner so that treatment if required can be commenced. Incidence rates reflect that in 3–5/1000 live births may require a Pavlik Harness and 1–2/1000 may require surgery.

The term 'developmental' reflects that this condition can develop any time between uterine life and into early childhood. DDH can have long-term sequelae such as impaired mobility, pain or osteoarthritis of the hip and back if it remains undetected or when treatment is delayed. Therefore, early detection, diagnosis and treatment can improve later health and reduce the need for surgical intervention. Assessment of neonatal instability of the hip is also complicated by its natural history of resolution, in that 60% of dislocatable hips will resolve, with 70–90% resolving spontaneously within the first few weeks.

Predisposing risk factors

In general, the key risk factors for DDH can be identified within the maternal and neonatal records and parents should always be asked if they have any concerns or any further information that may be useful. It is worth reading the research of Ionescu et al. (2023), who identified the most prevalent risk factors (which also included female infant and oligohydramnios) that they found during their retrospective study. However, in the UK the risk factors identified by the National Screening Committee (PHE, 2021a) are as follows:

• **First-degree relative**: either a parent or sibling of the baby who had a history of hip problems as a baby and needed treatment with a splint, harness or operation.
• **Breech presentation**: babies at ≥36 weeks' gestation, irrespective of the presentation at the time of delivery or the mode of delivery. This includes babies who have had a successful external cephalic version and those who have presented breech at the time of birth between 28 weeks' gestation and term. The breech presentation needs to be recorded as confirmed by the practitioner if they are sure of their findings or via USS. However, good observational skills can also detect those babies that have not been detected in the breech position antenatally; for example, a baby who has been lying in a frank breech position will often assume a position post birth where the legs are raised in the air.
• **Multiple birth**: all babies from a multiple pregnancy with any of the NIPE hip risk factors listed here should have a hip USS, as it may be difficult to accurately identify which baby was affected.

Examination process

The hip examination comprises three parts: investigation, observation and manipulation (Table 49.1). Observation commences from the moment the legs are visualised. Manipulation consists of both Ortolani and Barlow manoeuvres: the Ortolani manoeuvre is used to screen for a dislocated hip and Barlow is used to screen for a dislocatable hip (see Table 49.2).

Only a practitioner experienced in conducting the hip examination should perform the manoeuvres unless they are learning how to complete them, in which case they should be supervised while doing so. Both manoeuvres are for screening purposes only and generally the more experienced the practitioner, the easier and more effective the manoeuvres. Therefore, this brings into question whether junior doctors receive enough, appropriate training and supervision to enable them to detect anomalies.

The baby should be examined in a warm environment and on a firm, flat surface (the maternal bed flexes too much), as this will improve effectivity. Sometimes the assistance of a parent may be required to encourage the baby to suckle on a finger during the manoeuvres to aid in relaxation. The parent(s) should be informed that the manoeuvres used do not hurt the baby. However, the baby may become irritated when their legs are being held and because often this manoeuvre occurs at the end of the examination process. See Table 49.2 for an explanation of how these manoeuvres are performed.

The examination findings should be documented within the neonatal record, digital record and S4N system (if available) and in the PCHR. Any anomalies must be discussed with the neonatologist and the practitioner should be aware of local policy regarding referral (Tables 49.1 and 49.2 highlight the screen positive findings).

Examination findings

• **Screen negative examination, no risk factors**: No anomalies were found during the examination and no risk factors have been identified, so no further action is required. The next assessment will occur at 6 to 8 weeks with the GP and if no anomalies are found at this stage, the child will enter the Healthy Child Programme.
• **Screen negative examination, with risk factors**: Refer for hip ultrasound within 6 weeks. Babies with no predisposing risk factors but who are found to have 'clicky' hip (high-pitched click, usually ligamentous in origin) should be managed as per the local referral policy, as they are not included in the NIPE screening programme key performance data.
• **Screen positive**: One or more of the screen positive factors (PHE, 2021a), with or without the presence of risk factors, indicates the need for the baby to be referred to the neonatologist and attend for hip USS within the target timescales. Refer to the NIPE screening handbook (PHE, 2021a) for current information regarding gestational age, USS and clinical assessment by an orthopaedic specialist. Guidance is also given in the event that a hip rescan is required in order to reduce possible delay. Also, practitioners should be conversant with the NIPE newborn hip screening: screen positive pathway (PHE, 2021f). A baby found to be screen positive following the 6 to 8 week infant examination will be referred directly to an orthopaedic surgeon for urgent expert opinion, which should occur by 10 weeks of age.

Necessary information for parents

Parents need to be asked to observe their child's leg movement and if they have concerns at any time to contact their midwife, GP or health visitor. In particular, PHE (2021a) advocates that parents should observe for the following:

• One leg cannot be moved out sideways as far as the other when changing the baby's nappy.
• One leg seems to be longer than the other.
• One leg drags when their baby starts crawling.
• Their child walks with a limp or has a 'waddling' gait.

It is clear that the 'one-stop shop' model of integrated care, where initial and ongoing care (if required) is accessible within the same venue and at the same time, is regarded as the most effective provision of care.

Natural development of the hips is facilitated by practices that mimic the fetal flexed position, allowing plenty of hip movement, flexion and adduction. Conversely, an unhealthy position, when the legs are held in extension with the hips and knees straight and/ or when the legs are held together, inhibits hip development, raising the potential for misalignment and dislocation. Therefore, the importance of slings that promote flexion and abduction of the hip, car seats with a wide seat base allowing the legs to sit naturally apart and the baby not sitting in a car seat too long should be discussed with the parent(s). This also links with Box 35.1 in Chapter 35, which highlights activities that assist the baby's natural progression from involuntary to voluntary reflexes.

50 Genitalia: female

Figure 50.1 Normal female genitalia of newborn.

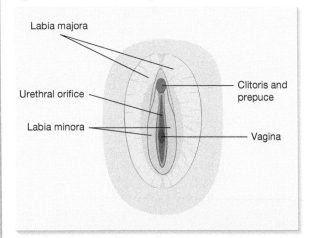

Labia majora

Urethral orifice

Labia minora

Clitoris and prepuce

Vagina

Figure 50.2 Inguinal hernia.

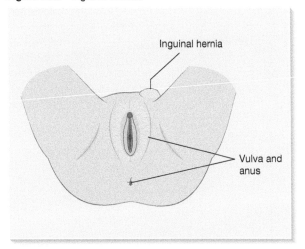

Inguinal hernia

Vulva and anus

Figure 50.3 Fusion of labia majora.

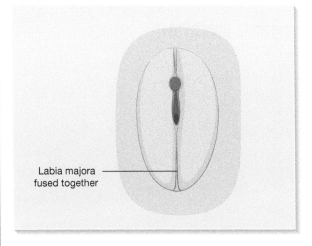

Labia majora fused together

Figure 50.4 Pseudo-menstruation (blood-stained, mucus discharge).

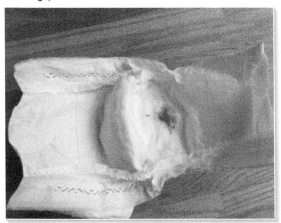

Figure 50.5 Urates (brick-coloured, powdery deposits).

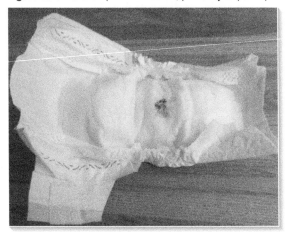

Figure 50.6 Ambiguous genitalia.

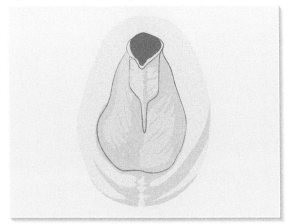

Physical Examination of the Newborn at a Glance, Second Edition. Dr Lyn Dolby and Denise (Dee) Campbell.
© 2025 John Wiley & Sons Ltd. Published 2025 by John Wiley & Sons Ltd.

The examination should take place in a warm environment with the groin and genitalia area clean and fully exposed. Inspection includes assessment of the groin, labia, clitoris, vagina, urethra and perineum (Figure 50.1). Palpation confirms the absence of any masses. Palpation of a normal bladder and confirmation of urine output are reassuring features. Appearance of anuria or oliguria up to 48 hours in an otherwise healthy infant may not be a concern if there is no palpable bladder, plus micturition may have been missed. Apply a urine collection bag and a tissue over the urethra to monitor. Risk factors from the full history are important, particularly ultrasound results. Cardiac anomalies, numbers of umbilical cord vessels, oligo- or polyhydramnios and musculoskeletal abnormalities all increase the risk of renal and genital anomalies.

Groin

The groin should be flat, without inflammation or swelling, even during crying (when intra-abdominal pressure increases). The femoral pulse should be palpable but not visible, except in a premature or significantly small for dates infant. The most common abnormalities can both occur at the same time:

- **Inguinal hernia** (Figure 50.2): bulging within the groin area is the most common hernia of the newborn. Incomplete closure of the processus vaginalis allows protrusion of uterus, fallopian tubes or intestines into the soft tissue and labia. The condition may be present at birth but more commonly develops in the first few weeks and should be soft, disappearing spontaneously during rest or able to be digitally reduced and returned to the abdominal cavity. Intestine permanently trapped is said to be 'incarcerated'. Enlargement, darkening and hardening of the swelling, accompanied by increasing pain and vomiting, may indicate strangulation (reduction of blood supply and tissue death).
- **Hydrocele**: a bulging, fluid-filled mass caused by peritoneal fluid within the processus vaginalis.

Labia

The labia majora are a normal skin colour and cover the labia minora at term. There should be no skin tags, adhesions or fusion between the two sides of the labia. The skin should not be tense and shiny or be covered in rugae. Some swelling is possible because of the effect of maternal hormones (lasts weeks) or trauma during breech birth (lasts days) and may be accompanied by bruising. The size should not appear disproportionately large or change along the length of each labia. Enlargement, rugae or a sack-like swelling arouses suspicion of ambiguous genitalia and indeterminate sex. Similarly, any masses need investigation as they could be one or more testes (ovaries do not descend), a mucoid cyst or, more rarely, a tumour.

You will need to gently separate the labia majora to inspect the labia minora. These are usually smaller, brighter coloured and appear moist. It is also likely that they will be covered in a cheesy white substance. This is vernix, which will be naturally absorbed over the first days of life. The most common abnormalities seen are as follow:

- **Adhesions** can be seen in otherwise normal infants.
- **Fusion** (Figure 50.3) may be adrenogenital syndrome or ambiguous genitalia.
- **Pigmentation** increases with ambiguous genitalia and strangulation of hernia.

Clitoris

The clitoris and prepuce (a shorter foreskin) are very prominent at birth (**cliteromegaly**) because of increased circulating hormones including increased androgen production. They protrude from the upper join of the labia minora. The most common abnormality is **bifid clitoris**: a split clitoris, often with no prepuce.

Vagina and urethra

The urethra lies directly below the clitoris but is rarely visible in the newborn unless there is an associated prolapse or cyst. Normal urine streams and a non-palpable bladder are reassuring features. The vaginal orifice should be easily visible below the clitoris, 1.5 cm in diameter and embedded between the pairs of labia. A white, mucoid blood-stained loss, associated with maternal hormones, may be evident (pseudo-menstruation; Figure 50.4). The most common abnormalities are as follows:

- **Epispadias**: the urethra lies above or to the side of the clitoris; commonly associated with an absent or bifid clitoris.
- **Hydrocolpos**: obstruction (possibly imperforate hymen) of the vagina with distension because of secretion build-up behind the obstruction.
- **Hydrometrocolpos**: hydrocolpos extended to the uterine cavity.
- **Hymenal tag**: thickened vascular membrane protruding from the vagina with a central orifice; common but resolves spontaneously.
- **Imperforate hymen**: hymen has no meatus. Bulges from the vagina after obstructing the vagina and with a build-up of secretions.
- **Urates** (Figure 50.5): a combination of calcium and urate crystals, formed during mild dehydration; passed in urine as a brown-pink powdery stain.
- **Urethral polyp**: interlabial protrusion with meatus that leaks urine; rarely obstructs in females.
- **Urogenital sinus/fistula**: dip or channel between urethra and uterus or vagina.
- **Vaginal skin tag**: benign skin growth around the vaginal orifice.

Perineum

Examine the perineum for dimpling, fistulae, skin tags, cysts and masses and to ensure that the anus is at least one fingertip away from the genitalia.

Ambiguous genitalia

Ambiguous genitalia may include some or all of the following: clitoral enlargement that looks phallic; fusion of the labia majora; an abnormally located urethral meatus; and/or a palpable mass (Figure 50.6). Increased virilisation (masculinisation) will have occurred. The cause for a female infant will be congenital adrenal hyperplasia (ACTH), when XX females develop masculinised (androgynous) genitalia following excessive production of testosterone. However, at birth the female status is not known and the infant should be referred to as 'baby' until the sex can be decided on. This decision will require involvement of the paediatrician, endocrinologist, geneticist and urologist. They will consider the genetic sex (chromosomal karyotype). gonadal sex (presence or absence of testes) and functional sex (possibilities with current organs), and screen for adrenal hyperplasia (ACTH, urea and electrolytes). If a mass is palpated this may be testes, as ovaries never descend into or below the groin.

51 Genitalia: male

Figure 51.1 Embryology of testicular descent.
Source: Lissauer et al. (2020) / John Wiley & Sons.

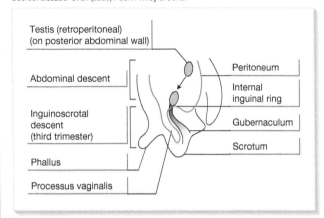

Figure 51.2 Normal obliterated processus vaginalis.
Source: Lissauer et al. (2020) / John Wiley & Sons.

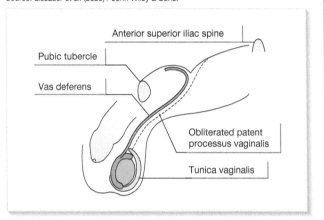

Figure 51.3 Inguinal hernia (widely patent processus vaginalis).
Source: Lissauer et al. (2020) / John Wiley & Sons.

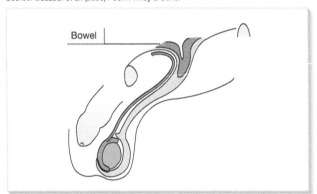

Figure 51.4 Hypospadias.
Source: Reproduced with permission from Lissauer et al. (2020) / John Wiley & Sons.

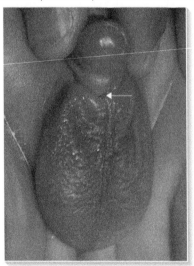

Figure 51.5 Classifications of hypospadias.
Source: Lissauer et al. (2020) / John Wiley & Sons.

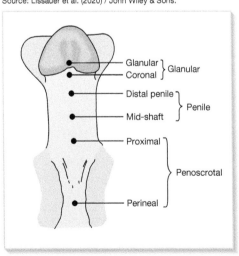

Figure 51.6 Hydrocele (narrowly patent processus vaginalis).
Source: Lissauer et al. (2020) / John Wiley & Sons.

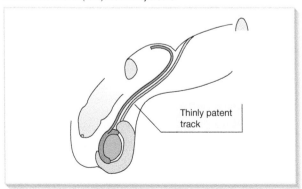

Physical Examination of the Newborn at a Glance, Second Edition. Dr Lyn Dolby and Denise (Dee) Campbell.
© 2025 John Wiley & Sons Ltd. Published 2025 by John Wiley & Sons Ltd.

The examination should take place in a warm environment with genitalia clean and exposed. Inspection is of the groin, penis, scrotal sac and perineum. Palpation confirms the presence (or absence) of the testes and any masses. The palpation of a normal bladder and confirmation of urine output are reassuring features. Anuria or oliguria (up to 48 hours) in an otherwise healthy infant may not be a concern if there is no palpable bladder, as micturition may have been missed. Apply a urine collection bag and a tissue over the urethra to monitor. Risk factors are considered including ultrasound results and family history: cardiac anomalies, numbers of umbilical cord vessels, oligo- or polyhydramnios and musculoskeletal abnormalities increase the risk of renal and genital anomalies.

Groin

The groin should not appear enflamed or swollen along the line of testicular descent (Figures 51.1 and 51.2) and not bulge even during crying (when intra-abdominal pressure increases). The femoral pulse should be palpable but not visible, except in a premature or significantly small for dates infant.

Inguinal hernia (Figure 51.3)

This is the most common abnormality and is seen as bulging within the groin area. Incomplete closure of the inguinal canal allows protrusion of intestines towards or into the scrotum. It may be present at birth but more often develops in the first weeks. It should be soft, disappearing spontaneously during rest or able to be digitally returned to the abdominal cavity. Intestine permanently trapped is said to be 'incarcerated'. Enlargement, darkening and hardening of the swelling, accompanied by increasing pain and vomiting, may indicate strangulation (reduction of blood supply and tissue death).

Penis

The penis should be straight and of normal skin tone, stretching to 3.5 cm from the pubic bone to the prepuce (foreskin) and glans and 1 cm wide mid-shaft. Pads of fat over the symphysis pubis can make it appear shorter (micropenis). The prepuce covers the head of the penis. It is not retractable (phimosis) for 2 years but should not be tight. The urethral meatus is a small orifice, typically visible centrally at the tip of the penis, allowing a straight, continuous urine flow. If the meatus is not visible but urine is passed from below the prepuce without it ballooning, this is reassuring – check there is no meatus visible elsewhere. The most common abnormalities of the penis are as follows:

- **Aphallia**: no penis.
- **Bifid penis**: two halves to penile shaft with one urethra; associated with cloacal exstrophy (exposure of abdominal organs and bladder).
- **Chordee**: over-developed fibrous tissue with traction and bend of the penis. Downward chordee can be associated with hypospadias.
- **Diphallia**: duplicated penis; bifid or true duplication.
- **Epispadias**: urethral meatus on upper aspect; extremely rare but may be as extreme as bladder exstrophy.
- **Hooded prepuce**: prepuce is absent on the underside of the glans. Common alongside hypospadias.
- **Hypospadias** (Figures 51.4 and 51.5): abnormal location of urethral meatus under penis, with incomplete urethra. Three types:
  - **Glanular** (coronal or balanic): at base of glans, may include hooded prepuce, shallow pit over end of penis, meatus at lower end of pit.
  - **Penile** (distal or midshaft): between glans and scrotum.
  - **Penoscrotal** (proximal and perineal): opens where penis and scrotum join or on the perineum.
- **Micropenis**: short and/or thin penis; beware ambiguous genitalia.

- **Posterior urethral valves**: congenital blockage within the urethra.
- **Priapism**: erections are normal and common.

Scrotum and testes

The scrotum should be symmetrical, slightly darker than the surrounding skin, covered in rugae, with a midline ridge. The testes are ovoid, firm, smooth and equal in size (1–1.5 cm). When palpating, resist the temptation to press directly onto the scrotum, as this can ballot the testis up along the inguinal canal. Instead, begin at the upper groin and, using two fingers, digitally palpate each side, down along the inguinal canal and into the scrotum until the testis is felt (or you are confident it is not within the scrotal sac). This part of the examination is assessing for unilateral or bilateral undescended testes, which affects 2–6% of term male newborns and is associated with a later risk of testicular cancer, reduced fertility, urogenital problems (e.g. hypospadias and testicular torsion), endocrine disorders or ambiguous genitalia (PHE, 2021a). Risk factors include being pre-term, small for gestation, low birth weight and a first-degree family history.

Cryptorchidism (unilateral or bilateral undescended testes)

Identification of unilateral undescended testis at the newborn assessment should be reassessed at the 6–8-week infant NIPE; bilateral undescended testes require review by a senior paediatrician within 24 hours for consideration of metabolic disorders and sex determination (PHE, 2021a,b,g). Persistent unilateral undescended testis at the 6–8-week examination requires a further review by the GP at 4–5 months and surgical review by a paediatrician before 6 months, but persistent bilateral undescended testes should be referred to a senior paediatrician within 2 weeks (PHE, 2021a,c,g).

The other abnormalities of the scrotum and testes are as follows:
- **Anorchia**: absence of both testes.
- **Bifid scrotum**: two separated scrotal sacs.
- **Bruising**: trauma; may be caused by breech presentation.
- **Ectopic testis**: starts to descend but stops, often at inguinal pouch.
- **Hydrocele** (Figure 51.6): fluid-filled scrotum.
- **Oedema**: as a result of hormones or trauma.
- **Pigmentation**: darkening of scrotum; may be a sign of congenital adrenal hyperplasia or torsion of the testes.
- **Smooth scrotum**: associated with anorchia and prematurity.
- **Testicular torsion**: twisted testes; reddened/darkened, swollen scrotum; does not transilluminate; leads to ischaemia and necrosis.
- **Webbed penis**: scrotal sack extends up penis and may reach glans.

Perineum

Confirm there is no additional meatus, fistula or mass and that normal spacing occurs between scrotum and anus.

Ambiguous genitalia

Ambiguous genitalia may result from the following:
- **Under-virilised male**: aphallia, micropenis, smooth scrotum, anorchia or ectopic testes, abnormally located urethra.
- **Virilised female**: cliteromegaly, labial fusion.
- **Ovotesticular disorder**: testicular and ovarian tissue present.

The infant should be referred to as 'baby' until the sex is confirmed. This will require involvement of a paediatrician, endocrinologists, geneticists and urologists, who will consider the genetic sex (chromosomal karyotype), gonadal sex (presence or absence of testes) and functional sex (possibilities with current organs), and screen for adrenal hyperplasia (ACTH, urea and electrolytes).

52 Lower limbs and feet

Figure 52.1   Normal anteriorly bowed and flexed legs.

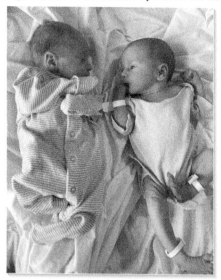

Figure 52.3   Newborn leg damaged by amniotic bands.
Source: Phänotyp / Wikimedia Commons / CC BY-SA 4.0.

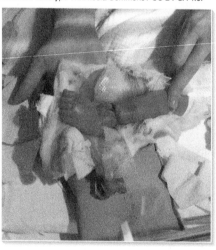

Figure 52.5   Normal creases.

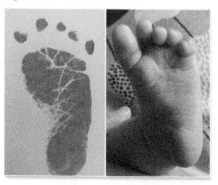

Figure 52.2   Positive Allis sign with unequal knee heights.

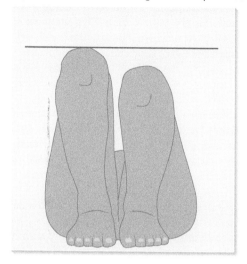

Figure 52.4   Congenital talipes varus.

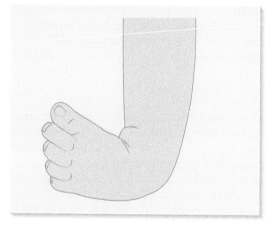

Figure 52.6   Deep plantar crease and wider space between toes (trisomy 21).

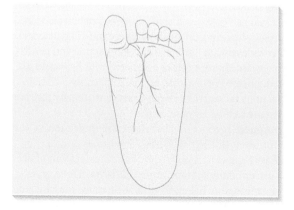

This chapter considers the legs and feet. Assessments of the hip and the reflexes are considered in their own chapters and will include assessment of gluteal leg folds. Abnormalities of the lower limbs and feet are associated with a range of causes, including genetic disorders and their resultant syndromes (e.g. achondroplasia and Marfan syndrome), hypocalcaemia (e.g. hypoparathyroidism) and amniotic bands. Assessment is of bones, joints and muscle and includes checking for symmetry of shape as well as range of movement across both legs.

Some conditions affect both the upper and lower limbs. Since 1962 and the withdrawal of thalidomide for pregnant women, the most common cause of multiple limb abnormalities, which may affect upper as well as lower limbs, is achondroplasia. **Achondroplasia (dwarfism)** and **Kniest dysplasia (disproportionate dwarfism)** are genetic conditions that involve reduced calcium and collagen, affecting all bone and joint development. The femur is shortened and bowed, joints are enlarged and the toes are short and fat.

Legs

The examination of the legs considers the femur, tibia, fibula, patella, soft tissue and musculature. The practitioner needs to be aware that the legs of a newborn will always appear slightly anteriorly bowed and flexed when at rest (Figure 52.1). Symmetry of the length of the legs should be assessed using the Allis sign (Figure 52.2). This involves the lower legs being bent, feet placed flat and equidistant from the midline, then observing the height of the knees to ensure symmetry – unequal heights are a positive Allis sign. Rare abnormalities include the following:

- **Amniotic bands** (Figure 52.3): a fibrous band from the amniotic sac tangles around the developing fetus, constricting blood supply and disturbing development. This may affect either upper or lower limbs and occasionally upper and lower at the same time.
- **Congenital femoral deficiency**: very rare; associated with shortening or absence of one or both femurs; may extend to tibias, fibulas and the patellae.
- **Dislocated knee**: various degrees of extension of the knee are seen, requiring manipulation to stabilise. Often found in association with DDH and talipes.
- **Dislocated patella**: the patella has moved laterally. This injury is often missed and may occur with trisomy 21.
- **Fractures**: rare, but should be considered following a traumatic birth, particularly breech extraction. Signs and symptoms of fracture include asymmetrical shape, reduced mobility, pain, irregularities along the bone, bruising or haematoma, crepitus, and a callus forming 7–10 days after delivery. Crepitus will be felt (and may be heard) as a grating sensation where the two ends of the fractured bone meet. However, most lower-limb fractures are avulsion fractures, caused when a ligament or muscle is over-stretched during traumatic delivery, causing the snapping of a small part of the epiphysis away from the main bone.
- **Limb-reduction defects**: affect upper or lower limbs and occasionally both at the same time. This is when part of, or the whole of, a limb fails to develop fully.
- **Nail-patella syndrome**: on examination, the nails are absent or poorly formed and there will be an indentation rather than a curvature over the patella bone of the knee. The knees may turn inwards and movement is limited; assessment may reveal small or missing patellae.

- **Sirenomelia (mermaid syndrome)**: extremely rare; affecting the spine, pelvis, lower limbs, genitals and lower abdomen (plus internal organs). The newborn has full or partial fusion of the legs. Foot abnormalities include no feet, one foot or backwards-facing feet.
- **Tumours**: very rare; may be deeper within the leg or on the skin (e.g. haemangioma). Any unusual lump or swelling should be investigated.

Feet and ankles

- **Talipes**: the most common mild abnormality related to the feet and ankles, when one or both feet turn inwards (invert). It results from constriction in utero and reduced joint movement. Gentle pressure on the outer side of the soles of the feet enables normal positioning without any discomfort for the newborn. Forms of congenital talipes that cannot be gently reduced, affect one or both feet and may combine two types in one deformity are:
  - **Talipes calcaneus**: when the foot pulls up towards the shin at the ankle (dorsiflexion).
  - **Talipes cavus**: a high-arched foot.
  - **Talipes equinus**: the foot angles away from the shin at the ankle and points downwards.
  - **Talipes valgus**: the foot is abducted and everted, and twisted outwards.
  - **Talipes varus** (Figure 52.4): the foot is adducted and inverted, and twisted inwards. Positional talipes varus is seen in Figure 52.1.
- **Rocker-bottom feet**: the heel (calcaneus) is prominent and the talus (ankle bone) has developed further along the foot, creating a convex sole. This abnormality is associated with many neuromuscular and chromosomal abnormalities (e.g. trisomy 18).
- **Simian crease** (Figures 52.5 and 52.6): a deeply grooved plantar crease running longitudinally from between the big toe and the second toe. Commonly associated with genetic conditions such as trisomy 21, but can occasionally occur in genetically normal newborns.

Toes

Many of the abnormalities of the toes are similar to those of the fingers:

- **Absent or deformed nails**: may also have nail-patella syndrome.
- **Arachnodactyly (spider legs)**: unusually long toes. Associated with connective tissue disorders (e.g. Marfan syndrome).
- **Brachydactyly**: short toes.
- **Camptodactyly**: one or more abnormally bent toes; fixed flexion.
- **Clinodactyly**: a curving toe; may cause overlapping.
- **Macrodactyly**: one or more enlarged toes.
- **Oligodactyly**: one or more absent toes.
- **Polydactyly**: one or more extra toes.
- **Sandal gap**: wide space between first and big toe (can be associated with trisomy 21).
- **Short, fat toes**: seen in achondroplasia and hypoparathyroidism.
- **Symbrachdactyly**: short toes, plus webbing.
- **Syndactyly**: fused toes; may be at skin level or include bone.
- **Webbing**: this may be reduced (limiting movement) or increased (either extending up the length of the toe or as excessive folds).

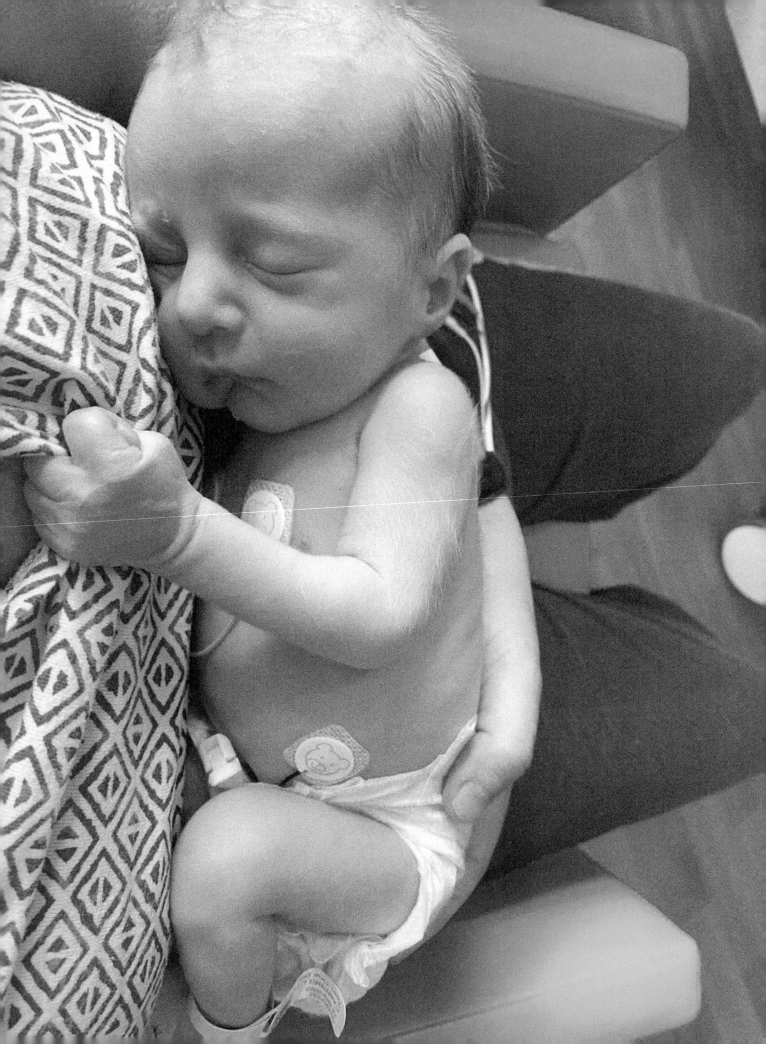

Revision and self-assessment

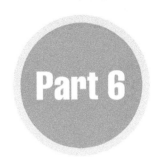

Part 6

Chapters

53 Self-test crosswords

These two crosswords provide an opportunity to test your knowledge and understanding. You will find the answers on page 129.

Crossword 1

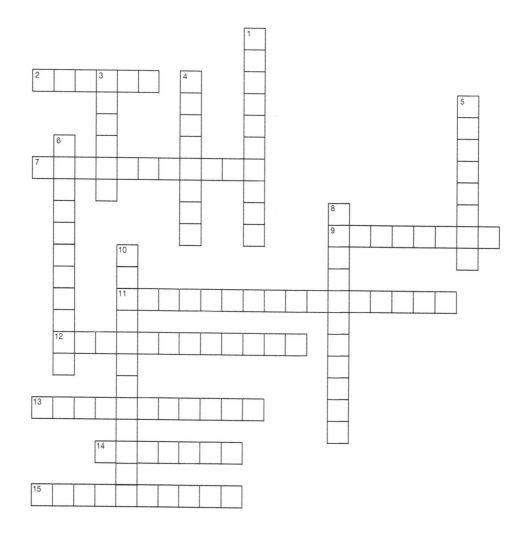

Across

2 The fontanelle that is found at the junction of the parietal and occipital bones.
7 A cold baby is experiencing this.
9 This manoeuvre tests for a dislocated hip.
11 The soft oedematous patch that may be found on the neonatal head due to pressure during labour.
12 Blue colouration of the neonatal hands and feet.
13 Herniation of abdominal contents into the umbilical cord, encapsulated by a clear sac.
14 Ventral curvature of the penis.
15 Term used for fused digits.

Down

1 In undescended testes there is an increased risk of this.
3 This manoeuvre tests for a dislocatable hip.
4 Most common eye condition in neonates.
5 Sound caused by expiration through a partially closed glottis.
6 Abnormal placement of the urethral meatus on the underside of the penis.
8 One or more extra digits.
10 An abnormally small chin.

Crossword 2

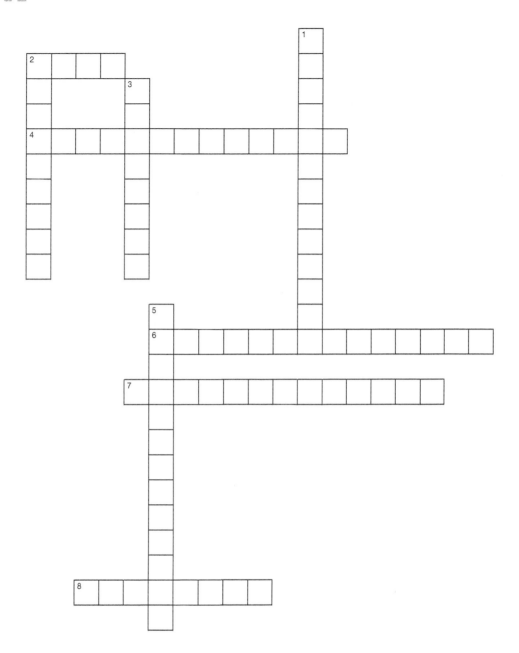

Across

2 Abbreviation for sudden infant death syndrome.
4 Inability to breakdown galactose into glucose.
6 Instrument used to assess the fundal (red) reflex.
7 The condition when the blood sugar concentration drops below a predetermined level.
8 Reflex that usually occurs after plantar flexion has been elicited.

Down

1 Jaundice that usually occurs at around 3–4 days post birth.
2 Another name for subaponeurotic haemorrhage.
3 Green-black stool evacuated from the bowel during the first 2–3 days of life.
5 The condition resulting from excessive red blood cells or high packed cell volume.

54 Self-test multiple-choice questions

The following multiple-choice questions provide a self-test quiz for you to check your knowledge and understanding. You will find the answers on page 129.

1 **How long** does it take for the transformation from fetal to neonatal circulation to be completed?
  (a) 24 hours
  (b) 4 days
  (c) 1 month
  (d) 6 weeks

2 Transient neonatal tachypnoea can occur in the newborn but is normally mild and resolves in a few days. What is the **percentage** of babies in which this condition occurs?
  (a) 1%
  (b) 2%
  (c) 3%
  (d) 4%

3 An infant of a mother with diabetes can be at greater risk of **which one** of the following?
  (a) Macrosomia
  (b) Respiratory distress syndrome
  (c) Polycythaemia
  (d) All of the above

4 **How** is 'harlequin' colour change in a baby exhibited?
  (a) Blueness around the mouth of the neonate
  (b) Mottling of the skin
  (c) Feet are blue but hands remain well perfused
  (d) A clear, demarcated line of redness and an area of paleness that divides the neonate from head to abdomen

5 **Which one** of the following gives the measurement for the anterior fontanelle?
  (a) 1 cm × 1 cm
  (b) 3.4 cm × 1.5 cm
  (c) 6.1 cm × 3 cm
  (d) 3 cm × 3 cm

6 Physiological jaundice is due to **which one** of the following?
  (a) Infection
  (b) ABO incompatibility
  (c) Natural breakdown of excess red blood cells
  (d) Rhesus isoimmunisation

7 A normal newborn rash is often seen in the term neonate during the first week of life. Which term is **correct**?
  (a) Vernix caseosa
  (b) Erythema toxicum neonatorum
  (c) Naevus flammeus
  (d) None of the above

8 What is the approximate **ratio** of hyperpigmented macule in dark-skinned and pale-skinned babies?
  (a) 70% : 10%
  (b) 50% : 50%
  (c) 50% : 30%
  (d) 40% : 30%

9 The neonate is more likely to become jaundiced in certain circumstances. Which one of the following reasons is **incorrect**?
  (a) Slow evacuation of meconium
  (b) The presence of bruising resulting from pressure during labour or birth trauma
  (c) Infection
  (d) Adequate levels of fluid intake

10 Which of the following is **not** considered to be a neurological alarm signal?
  (a) Persistent irritability
  (b) Bilateral and equal Moro reflex
  (c) Hypotonia
  (d) Abnormal cry

11 A healthy term neonate is capable of demonstrating a number of reflexes at birth. Which one of the following is **not** a reflex?
  (a) Rooting
  (b) Asymmetrical tonic neck
  (c) Asymmetrical eye movement
  (d) Moro

12 **Which one** of the following refers to the shiny, white spots found in the neonatal mouth or on the male genitalia?
  (a) Milia
  (b) Erythema neonatorum toxicum
  (c) Epstein pearls
  (d) Staphylococcal blisters

13 The foreskin of the penis can be retracted at **what age?**
  (a) From birth
  (b) Between 3 and 10 years of age
  (c) From 16 years of age
  (d) Not until 12 years of age

14 **Which one** of the following is a classic sign of Erb's palsy following a brachial plexus injury at birth?
  (a) Torticollis
  (b) Flexed arms
  (c) Waiter's tip posture
  (d) Arms are permanently flexed

15 A hemifacial port wine stain may be indicative of **which one** of the following conditions?
  (a) Trisomy 21
  (b) Sturge-Weber syndrome
  (c) Turner syndrome
  (d) Trisomy 18

16 **What** is the term for a serious condition arising from jaundice?
  (a) Encephalitis
  (b) Sheehan disease
  (c) Kernicterus
  (d) Thrombophilia

Physical Examination of the Newborn at a Glance, Second Edition. Dr Lyn Dolby and Denise (Dee) Campbell.
© 2025 John Wiley & Sons Ltd. Published 2025 by John Wiley & Sons Ltd.

55 Self-test crosswords and multiple-choice questions: answers

Crosswords

Crossword 1

Across
2 Lambda
7 Hypothermia
9 Ortolani
11 Caput succedaneum
12 Acrocyanosis
13 Omphalocele
14 Chordee
15 Syndactyly

Down
1 Malignancy
3 Barlow
4 Cataract
5 Grunting
6 Hypospadias
8 Polydactyly
10 Micrognathia

Crossword 2

Across
2 SIDS
4 Galactosaemia
6 Ophthalmoscope
7 Hypoglycaemia
8 Babinski

Down
1 Physiological
2 Subgaleal
3 Meconium
5 Polycythaemia

Multiple-Choice Questions

1 (d) 6 weeks

2 (a) 1%

3 (d) All of the above

4 (d) A clear, demarcated line of redness and an area of paleness that divides the neonate from head to abdomen

5 (b) 3.4 cm × 1.5 cm

6 (c) Natural breakdown of excess red blood cells

7 (b) Erythema toxicum neonatorum

8 (a) 70% : 10%

9 (d) Adequate levels of fluid intake

10 (b) Bilateral and equal Moro reflex

11 (c) Asymmetrical eye movement

12 (c) Epstein pearls

13 (b) Between 3 and 10 years of age

14 (c) Waiter's tip posture

15 (b) Sturge-Weber syndrome

16 (c) Kernicterus

Physical Examination of the Newborn at a Glance, Second Edition. Dr Lyn Dolby and Denise (Dee) Campbell.
© 2025 John Wiley & Sons Ltd. Published 2025 by John Wiley & Sons Ltd.

56 Professional reflection: knowledge and insight

When reading each scenario in this chapter, make sure that you are conversant with your local NHS Trust and national guidelines, as some scenarios will require you to have an understanding of these. However, you also need to critically analyse the guidelines, bearing in mind the research on which the guidance was originally based and whether it is due to be updated. Also explore the available related literature to see how this compares with the guidance. Whether you are a student or a qualified practitioner, it is your responsibility to be able to demonstrate an appreciation of the latest research if your professional practice is to be evidence based.

These scenarios aim to assist you to reflect on your level of practice and depth of understanding, plus how effectively you communicate and collaborate with other professionals and the parents for whom you are caring. Ask yourself whether there are gaps in the service provision in the NHS Trust within which you practise, and what actions or services you see as making a positive difference to your colleagues and parents/babies.

No answers have been provided for these scenario situations. We want to help you think about your particular geographical region in terms of the needs of the sample group of parents and babies that you come across, how positive collaboration and respect between disciplines are encouraged and whether changes need to be made.

1 In relation to babies with a darker-pigmented skin, how do you effectively assess for cyanosis, jaundice and fundal reflex?

2 Thinking of past experiences, to what extent have you taken into account the importance of investigating family, maternal and postnatal history prior to examining a baby?

3 A parent wishes to go home an hour after the birth of their baby and they want the NIPE to be conducted before discharge. What do you need to think about at this point in time, and in particular what information will you need to particularly emphasise to the parent in relation to the cardiovascular assessment?

4 How would you recognise neonatal infection? When was the last time you looked at the latest guidance relating to group B *Streptococcus*?

5 Do you understand what happens during hearing screening and what the equipment used assesses for? Are you aware of the information given to parents? Can the ward environment and behaviour of staff have an impact on the screening process?

6 A baby is 5 days old and appears to be jaundiced, is sleepy and not feeding well. What actions might you perform? How would you know whether this jaundice has a pathological cause?

7 How would you recognise a subaponeurotic (or subgaleal) haemorrhage and why is early recognition important?

8 Do you understand what SIDS and SUDI mean?

9 When are parents most receptive to information relating to health promotion and issues such as signs of neonatal ill health?

10 Are you up to date with the conditions that newborn blood spot screening tests for? Have you checked recently whether any new conditions are going to be added to the list?

11 If you are a NIPE practitioner, how do you ensure that your knowledge and skills are up to date? If you are a student, what updating provisions or expectations are you aware of?

12 How does knowledge of the 'energy triangle' assist you in recognising babies who are at risk of hypoglycaemia and hypothermia?

13 Do you know what is included in and what is different between the 'initial' and 'daily' newborn examinations?

14 What information would you provide regarding neonatal skin care and is it up to date? Do you give a rationale for the information you are giving to parents?

15 You watch a colleague performing the NIPE on a neonate without removing the nappy. What concerns does this raise for you?

16 You are examining a newborn and consider that the baby is less responsive and more hypotonic than might be typically expected. Would this be considered normal under certain circumstances and when would it raise concerns?

17 The mother of the baby you are examining mentions a family history of trisomy 21 and that she did not want any diagnostic tests to be performed during pregnancy. What are the reassuring or concerning features you might identify during the examination?

18 The parents state that their newborn baby vomits after every feed. What further information do you need and how does this vomiting specifically influence your thinking and actions?

19 How can you tell the difference between the Moro reflex, jitteriness and a seizure?

20 What is the rationale and information you should give parents about the use of car seats and baby slings?

21 The baby you are examining has a blue-grey discolouration apparent on the skin. What is the relevance of this, what do you need to think about and what actions might you need to take?

Physical Examination of the Newborn at a Glance, Second Edition. Dr Lyn Dolby and Denise (Dee) Campbell.
© 2025 John Wiley & Sons Ltd. Published 2025 by John Wiley & Sons Ltd.

References

Alsaeed AA. (2021) Surgical management of congenital pseudoarthrosis of the clavicle: Review of current concepts. *Cureus*, **13** (10), e18482. doi: https://doi.org/10.7759/cureus.18482.

Anthony R and McKinlay C. (2022) Adaptation for life after birth: A review of neonatal physiology. *Neonatal Anaesthesia*, **24** (1), 1–9.

Auerbach N, Gupta G and Mahajan K. (2023) Cystic hygroma. In *StatPearls*. StatPearls Publishing: Treasure Island, FL. https://www.ncbi.nlm.nih.gov/books/NBK560672 (accessed February 2024).

Aylott M. (2006) The neonatal energy triangle. Part 1: Metabolic adaptation. *Paediatric Nursing*, **18** (6), 38–42.

Bhattacharya, B., Baba, Y., Al Kabbani, A. et al. (2023). Cleidocranial dysostosis. *Radiopaedia*, 29 June. https://doi.org/10.53347/RId-10472

Birthrights (2024). Social services and maternity care. https://www.birthrights.org.uk/factsheets/social-services-and-maternity-care (accessed February 2024).

Brazelton T and Nugent K. (2011) *Neonatal Behavioural Assessment Scale* (4th edn). McKeith Press, London.

British Association of Perinatal Medicine (2024) *Newborn Early Warning Trigger and Track 2 [NEWTT 2] chart. Deterioration of the newborn. A framework for practice.* London: British Association of Perinatal Medicine. https://www.bapm.org/resources/deterioration-of-the-newborn-newtt-2-a-framework-for-practice (accessed February 2024).

Brosansky BS, Riley MM and Bogen DL. (2021) Neonatology, in *Zittelli and Davis' Atlas of Pediatric Diagnosis* (8th edn) (eds SC McIntyre, AJ Nowalk, J Garrison and BJ Zitelli) (pp. 43–70). Elsevier Saunders, Philadelphia, PA.

Carrasco M and Stafstrom CE. (2024) Neonatal seizures, in *Principles of Neonatology*. (eds. A Maheshwari) (pp. 427–437). Philadelphia, PA: Elsevier. https://doi.org/10.1016/B978-0-323-69415.00049-7.

Care Quality Commission (2024) Culturally appropriate care. https://www.cqc.org.uk/guidance-providers/adult-social-care/culturally-appropriate-care (accessed May 2024).

Centers for Disease Control and Prevention (CDC). (2024). Facts about cleft lip and cleft palate. https://www.cdc.gov/ncbddd/birthdefects/cleftlip.html (accessed February 2024).

Children Act (2004), c. 31. https://www.legislation.gov.uk/ukpga/2004/31/pdfs/ukpga_20040031_en.pdf (accessed February 2024).

Department for Education (2023). Children in need: 2022 to 2023. https://www.gov.uk.government/statistics/children-in-need-2022-2023 (accessed February 2024).

Department for Education (2024). Children's social care: National framework. https://www.gov.uk/government/publications/childrens-social-care-national-framework (accessed February 2024).

Department of Health (Northern Ireland) (2023). *Children's social care statistics for Northern Ireland. 2022/23.* https://www.health-ni.gov.uk/news/childrens-social-care-statistics-northern-ireland-202223 (accessed February 2024).

Diaz de Ortiz, L.E.D., and Mendez, M.D. (2023). Palatal and gingival cysts of the newborn. In *StatPearls*. Treasure Island, FL: StatPearls Publishing. https://www.ncbi.nlm.nih.gov/books/NBK493177/ (accessed February 2024).

Dolby, E. (2023) The influence of the working environment on midwifery staff and students in relation to the newborn and infant physical examination (NIPE). https://uhra.herts.ac.uk/handle/2299/27317 (accessed January 2024).

Ely, D.M. and Driscoll, A.K. (2019). Infant mortality in the United States, 2017: Data from the period linked birth/infant death file. Atlanta, GA: Centers for Disease Control and Prevention. https://stacks.cdc.gov/view/cdc/80304 (accessed February 2024).

Fanning B. (2024) Neurological assessment, in *Tappero and Honeyfield's Physical Assessment of the Newborn: A Comprehensive Approach to the Art of Physical Examination* (7th edn) (eds. CL Witt and CL Wallman). Springfield, IL: Springfield Publishing, ch. 12.

General Medical Council (2012). Professional standards: Protecting children and young people. https://www.gmc-uk.org/-/media/documents/protecting-children-and-young-people---english-20200114_pdf-48978248.pdf (accessed February 2024).

Goldsmith L, Robert A, Flohr C, Boyle R, Ussher M and Perkin MR. (2023) Routine infant skincare advice in the UK: A cross-sectional survey. *Clinical & Experimental Allergy*, **54** (1), 56–60.

González-García I, Urisarri A, Nogueiras R, Diéguez C, Couce M and López M. (2022) An updated view on human neonatal thermogenesis. *Nature Reviews: Endocrinology*, **18**, 263–264.

Hashmi HM, Shamim N, Kumar V, Anjum N and Ahmad K. (2021) Clavicular fractures in newborns: what happens to one of the commonly injured bones at birth? *Cureus*, **13** (9), e18372. https://doi.org/10.7759/cureus.18372.

Hawdon JM, Beer J, Sharp D. et al. (2017) Neonatal hypoglycaemia: learning from claims *Archives of Disease in Childhood. Fetal Neonatal Edition*, **102** (2), F110–F115.

Hay W. (2022) Symptomatic or asymptomatic neonatal hypoglycemia – can one tell the difference? *Journal of Pediatrics*, **245**, 7–9. https://doi.org/10.1016/j.jpeds.2022.03.044

HM Government (2023). *Working Together to Safeguard Children: A Guide to Multiagency Working to Help, Protect and Promote the Welfare of Children.* HMSO, London. https://assets.publishing.service.gov.uk/media/669e7501ab418ab055592a7b/Working_together_to_safeguard_children_2023.pdf (accessed August 2024).

ICON (2023). Babies cry, you can cope. https://iconcope.org (accessed February 2024).

Ionescu. A., Dragomirescu. M., Herdea. A. and Ulici. A. (2023) Developmental dysplasia of the hip: How many risk factors are needed? *Children*, **10**, 968. https://doi.org/10.3390/children10060968

Irvine, A., Hoeger, P., and Yan, A. (eds) (2011). *Harper's Textbook of Pediatric Dermatology*, 3e. Oxford: Blackwell.

Kelleher MM., Cro S., Van Vogt E., et al. (2021) Skincare interventions in infants for preventing eczema and food allergy: A Cochrane systematic review and individual data meta-analysis. *Clinical Experimental Allergy*, **52** (3), 402–418.

Khanmohammadi R, Mir F, Baniebrahimi G and Mirzaei H (2018) Oral tumors in children: diagnosis and management. *Journal of Cell Biochemistry*, **119** (3), 2474–2483. https://doi.org/10.1002/jcb.26316.

Kinsler, V. (2023). Congenital melanocytic naevus. Rickmansworth: Primary Care Dermatology Society. https://www.pcds.org.uk/clinical-guidance/congenital-melanocytic-naevus (accessed January 2024).

Kirk A, Webb A, Rodriguez-Prado Y and Dorotan-Guevara M. (2022) Newborn pulse oximetry screening: A review. *Progress in Pediatric Cardiology*, **65**, 101506. https://doi.org/10.1016/j.ppedcard.2022.101506

Physical Examination of the Newborn at a Glance, Second Edition. Dr Lyn Dolby and Denise (Dee) Campbell.
© 2025 John Wiley & Sons Ltd. Published 2025 by John Wiley & Sons Ltd.

Knittel, R. and Ardakani, N.M. (2023). Skin nonmelanocytic tumor. PathologyOutlines.com. https://www.pathologyoutlines.com/topic/skintumornonmelanocyticnevussebaceus.html (accessed January 2024).

Krawiec, C. and Muzio, M.R. (2023). Neonatal seizure. In *StatPearls*. Treasure Island, FL: StatPearls Publishing. https://www.ncbi.nlm.nih.gov/books/NBK554535 (accessed February 2024).

Kyokan M, Bochaton N, Jirapaet V and Pfister R. (2023) Early detection of cold stress to prevent hypothermia: a narrative review. *Sage Open Medicine*, **11**, 1–11.

Lakhani N, Kulkarni K, Barwell J, Vasudevan P and Dorkins H. (2024). *Clinical Genetics and Genomics at a Glance*. Wiley-Blackwell, Chichester.

Lissauer, T., and Fanaroff, A.A. (2011) *Neonatology at a Glance*, 2e. Oxford: Blackwell.

Lissauer, T and Fanaroff, A. (2011) *Neonatology at a Glance* ? (2nd edn). Oxford. Wiley Blackwell

Lissauer T, Fanaroff AA, Miall L and Fanaroff J. (2020) *Neonatology at a Glance* (4th edn). Wiley-Blackwell, Chichester.

Lissenkova S, Ugochinyere VU, Sid J., et al. (2022) Racial and ethnic disparities in the perinatal health of infants conceived by ART. *Pediatrics*, **150** (5), e2021055855. https://doi.org/10.1542/peds.2021-055855

Lullaby Trust, The (2020) Care of Next Infant (CONI). https://www.lullabytrust.org.uk/bereavement-support/how-we-can-support-you/our-care-of-next-infant-scheme (accessed August 2024).

Macorano E., Gentile M., Stellacci G. et al. (2023) 'Compressed baby head': A new 'abusive head trauma' entity? *Children*, **10** (1003), 1–13.

Maternal Mental Health Alliance (2023) The maternal mental health experiences of young mums. https://maternalmentalhealthalliance.org/media/filer_public/2b/c1/2bc1d7f4-b64e-40bc-96e3-ccf773c33ad0/final_-_the_maternal_mental_health_experiences_of_young_mums.pdf (accessed January 2024).

Matoba N and Collins Jr JW. (2017) Racial disparity in infant mortality. *Seminars in Perinatology* **41** (6), 354–359.

Modrell A and Tadi P. (2023) Primitive reflexes. In *StatPearls*. Treasure Island, FL: StatPearls Publishing. https://www.ncbi.nlm.nih.gov/books/NBK554606/ (accessed January 2024).

Muse Health (2021). How much bacteria is on your hands? https://www.musehealth.com/blogs/news/how-much-bacteria-is-on-your-hands (accessed February 2024).

NBCP (2022). Sudden unexpected death in infancy (SUDI) up to 12 months. National Bereavement Care Pathway. https://d8production.default.sands.uk0.bigv.io/sites/default/files/2022-08/NBCP%20SUDI%20short%20guidance%20July%202022.pdf (accessed August 2024).

NHS England (2019). NHS mental health implementation plan 2019/20 – 2023/2024. https://www.longtermplan.nhs.uk/wp-content/uploads/2019/07/nhs-mental-health-implementation-plan-2019-20-2023-24.pdf (accessed January 2024).

NHS England (2020). Uniforms and workwear: Guidance for NHS employers. https://www.england.nhs.uk/publication/uniforms-and-workwear-guidance-for-nhs-employers (accessed February 2024).

NHS England (2021). Involving and supporting partners and other family members in specialist perinatal mental health services: Good practice guide. https://www.england.nhs.uk/wp-content/uploads/2021/03/Good-practice-guide-March-2021.pdf (accessed January 2024).

NHS England (2022). NHS helps thousands of pregnant smokers kick the habit. https://www.england.nhs.uk/2022/07/nhs-helps-thousands-of-pregnant-smokers-kick-the-habit (accessed January 2024).

NHS England (2023a). Newborn and infant physical examination: training requirements. https://www.england.nhs.uk/long-read/newborn-and-infant-physical-examination-training-requirements (accessed January 2024).

NHS England (2023b). NHS long term workforce plan. https://www.england.nhs.uk/wp-content/uploads/2023/06/nhs-long-term-workforce-plan-v1.2.pdf (accessed January 2024).

NHS England (2023c). Three year delivery plan for maternity and neonatal services. https://www.england.nhs.uk/wp-content/uploads/2023/03/B1915-three-year-delivery-plan-for-maternity-and-neonatal-services-march-2023.pdf (accessed January 2024).

NHS England (2024). National infection prevention and control manual for England. https://www.england.nhs.uk/publication/national-infection-prevention-and-control (accessed January 2024).

NICE (2017a). Child abuse and neglect. NICE guideline [NG76]. National Institute for Health and Care Excellence. https://www.nice.org.uk/guidance/NG76 (accessed February 2024).

NICE (2017b). Healthcare-associated infections: prevention and control in primary and community care. Clinical guideline [CG 139]. National Institute for Health and Care Excellence. https://www.nice.org.uk/guidance/cg139/chapter/recommendations (accessed February 2024).

NICE (2023a). Jaundice in newborn babies under 28 days. Clinical guideline [CG98]. National Institute for Health and Care Excellence. https://www.nice.org.uk/guidance/cg98 (accessed February 2024).

NICE (2023b). Intrapartum care. NICE guideline [NG235]. National Institute for Health and Care Excellence. https://www.nice.org.uk/guidance/ng235/chapter/Recommendations#care-throughout-labour-in-all-birth-settings (accessed February 2024).

NMC (2018). *The Code*. London: Nursing and Midwifery Council. https://www.nmc.org.uk/standards/code (accessed February 2024).

NMC (2019). *Standards of Proficiency for Midwives*. London: Nursing and Midwifery Council. https://www.nmc.org.uk/globalassets/sitedocuments/standards/standards-of-proficiency-for-midwives.pdf (accessed February 2024).

Nutfilloyevna OD and Shokir qizi QM. (2024) Anatomical and physiological features of the skin structure in childhood. *American Journal of Pediatric Medicine and Health Sciences*, **2** (2), 25–32.

Odd D, Williams T, Stoianova S., et al. (2023) Newborn health and child mortality across England. *JAMA Network Open*, **6** (10), e2338055.

OHID (2021). Newborn and infant physical examination screening pathway requirements specification. Office for Health Improvement & Disparities. https://www.gov.uk/government/publications/newborn-and-infant-physical-examination-screening-pathway-requirements-specification/newborn-and-infant-physical-examination-screening-pathway-requirements-specification (accessed January 2024).

ONS (2023). Unexplained deaths in infancy, England and Wales: 2021. Office for National Statistics. https://www.ons.gov.uk/peoplepopulationandcommunity/birthsdeathsandmarriages/deaths/bulletins/unexplaineddeathsininfancyenglandandwales/2021 (accessed December 2023).

Pachego, D. and Singh, A. (2023). Benign neonatal sleep myoclonus. Sleep Foundation. https://sleepfoundation.org/baby-sleep/benign-neonatal-sleep-myoclonus (accessed February 2024).

Pease A, Turner N, Ingram J. et al. (2023) Changes in background characteristics and risk factors among SIDS infants in England: Cohort comparisons from 1993 to 2020. *British Medical Journal Open* 13: e076751. https://doi.org/10.1136/bmjopen-2023-076751.

Phalke, N. and Goldman, J.J. (2023). Cleft palate. In *StatPearls*. Treasure Island, FL: StatPearls Publishing. https://www.ncbi.nlm.nih.gov/books/NBK563128 (accessed February 2024).

PHE (2017). Newborn pulse oximetry screening pilot update. *PHE Screening*. Public Health England. https://phescreening.blog.gov.uk/2017/01/10/newborn-pulse-oximetry-screening-pilot-update (accessed February 2024).

PHE (2019). Guidelines for surveillance and audiological referral for infant and children following newborn hearing screen. Public Health England. https://www.gov.uk/government/publications/surveillance-and-audiological-referral-guidelines/guidelines-for-surveillance-and-audiological-referral-for-infants-and-children-following-newborn-hearing-screen (accessed February 2024).

PHE (2021a). Newborn and infant physical examination (NIPE) screening programme handbook. Public Health England. https://www.gov.uk/government/publications/newborn-and-infant-physical-examination-programme-handbook/newborn-and-infant-physical-examination-screening-programme-handbook (accessed January 2024).

PHE (2021b). Newborn and infant physical examination (NIPE) newborn screening pathway. Public Health England. https://www.gov.uk/government/publications/newborn-and-infant-physical-examination-programme-handbook/newborn-and-infant-physical-examination-nipe-newborn-screening-pathway (accessed January 2024).

PHE (2021c). Newborn and infant physical examination (NIPE) infant screening pathway. Public Health England. https://www.gov.uk/government/publications/newborn-and-infant-physical-examination-programme-handbook/newborn-and-infant-physical-examination-nipe-infant-screening-pathway (accessed January 2024).

PHE (2021d). NIPE newborn eye screening: screen positive pathway. Public Health England. https://www.gov.uk/government/publications/newborn-and-infant-physical-examination-programme-handbook/nipe-newborn-eye-screening-screen-positive-pathway (accessed January 2024).

PHE (2021e). NIPE newborn heart screening: Screen positive pathway. Public Health England. https://www.gov.uk/government/publications/newborn-and-infant-physical-examination-programme-handbook/nipe-newborn-heart-screening-screen-positive-pathway (accessed January 2024).

PHE (2021f). NIPE newborn hip screening: Screen positive pathway. Public Health England. https://www.gov.uk/government/publications/newborn-and-infant-physical-examination-programme-handbook/nipe-newborn-hip-screening-screen-positive-pathway (accessed January 2024).

PHE (2021g). NIPE newborn testes screening: Screen positive pathway. Public Health England. https://www.gov.uk/government/publications/newborn-and-infant-physical-examination-programme-handbook/nipe-newborn-testes-screening-screen-positive-pathway (accessed January 2024).

PHE (2021h). S4N: What to do if it's unavailable. Public Health England. https://www.gov.uk/government/publications/newborn-and-infant-physical-examination-nipe-national-it-system-what-to-do-if-its-unavailable/s4n-what-to-do-if-its-unavailable (accessed February 2024).

PHE (2022). Patient journey from screen to referral. Public Health England. https://www.gov.uk/government/publications/newborn-hearing-screening-programme-nhsp-operational-guidance/6-patient-journey-from-screen-to-referral (accessed February 2024).

Pisani F, Spagnoli C, Falsaperla R, Nagarajan L, Ramantani G. (2021) Seizures in the neonate: A review of etiologies and outcomes. *Seizure*, **85**, 48–56. https://doi.org/10.1016/j.seizure.2020.12.023.

Queremel Milani, D.A. and Tadi, P. (2024). Genetics, chromosome abnormalities. In *StatPearls*. Treasure Island, FL: StatPearls Publishing. https://ncbi.nlm.nih.gov/booksNBK557691 (accessed February 2024).

Rabe H, Gyte GM, Díaz-Rossello JL, Duley L. (2019) Effect of timing of umbilical cord clamping and other strategies to influence placental transfusion at preterm birth on maternal and infant outcomes. *Cochrane Database Systematic Reviews* **2019** (9): CD003248. https://doi.org/10.1002/14651858.CD003248.pub4

Regan K and Monnelly V. (2023) Introduction of newborn pulse oximetry screening (POS): Two-year outcomes and implications for practice. *Archives of Disease in Childhood*, **108**, A151–A152. https://doi.org/10.1155/2024/3279878

RCOG (2017). Maternal mental health: Women's voices. Royal College of Obstetricians and Gynaecologists. https://www.rcog.org.uk/media/3ijbpfvi/maternal-mental-health-womens-voices.pdf (accessed December 2023).

RCPCH (2016). Sudden unexpected death in infancy and childhood: Multi-agency guidelines for care and investigation. Royal College of Paediatrics and Child Health. https://www.rcpath.org/static/874ae50e-c754-4933-995a804e0ef728a4/Sudden-unexpected-death-in-infancy-and-childhood-2e.pdf (accessed January 2024).

RCPCH (2023). 'Think measles' poster. Royal College of Paediatrics and Child Health. https://www.rcpch.ac.uk/sites/default/files/2023-11/think-measles-poster-rcpch-rcgp-2023.pdf (accessed January 2024)

Resuscitation Council UK (2021). Newborn life support. https://www.resus.org.uk/sites/default/files/2021-05/Newborn%20Life%20Support%20Algorithm%202021.pdf (accessed February 2024).

Resuscitation Council UK, Fawke, J., Madar, J. et al. (2021a). Advanced resuscitation of the newborn infant. https://www.resus.org.uk/sites/default/files/2021-04/Advanced%20Resuscitation%20of%20the%20Newborn%20Infant%20Algorithm%202021.pdf (accessed February 2024).

Resuscitation Council UK, Fawke, J., Madar, J. et al. (2021b). Newborn resuscitation and support of transition of infants at birth guidelines. https://www.resus.org.uk/library/2021-resuscitation-guidelines/newborn-resuscitation-and-support-transition-infants-birth (accessed February 2024).

Roeper M, Hoermann H, Kummer S, and Meissner T. (2023) Neonatal hypoglycemia: Lack of evidence for a safe management. *Frontiers in Endocrinology*, **14**: 1179102. https://doi.org/10.3389/fendo.2023.1179102.

Rueda J, Gutierrez J, Facio J, et al. (2022) Human tail in a newborn. *Journal of Pediatric Surgery Case Reports*, **76**, 102098. https://doi.org/10.1016/j.epsc.2021.102098.

Scottish Government (2023). Children's social work statistics Scotland: 2021 to 2022. https://www.gov.scot/publications/childrens-social-work-statistics-scotland-2021-22 (accessed February 2024).

Sinha S, Miall L and Jardin L. (2018) *Essential Neonatal Medicine* (6th edn). Wiley-Blackwell, Oxford.

Thomas RK (2015). *Practical medical procedures at a glance.* John Wiley & Sons.

Tanous A, Watad M, Felszer-Fisch, C., et al. (2021) Risk factors for mortality among newborns with neonatal seizures. *Neuropediatrics*, **52** (2), 084–091. https://doi.org/10.1055/s-0040-1712487.

Thomson, K., Moffat, M., Arisa, A. et al. (2021). Socioeconomic inequalities and adverse pregnancy outcomes in the UK and Republic of Ireland: A systematic review and meta analysis. *BMJ Open* **11**(3): e042753. https://doi.org/10.1136/bmjopen-2020-042753

UK Health Security Agency (2023). A guide to immunisation for babies up to 13 months of age – from February 2022. https://www.gov.uk/government/publications/a-guide-to-immunisations-for-babies-up-to-13-months-of-age/a-guide-to-immunisation-for-babies-up-to-13-months-of-age-from-february-2022 (accessed January 2024).

UK Health Security Agency (2024). National measles guidelines. https://assets.publishing.service.gov.uk/media/65bb924dcc6fd600145dbe4d/20240123_national-measles-guidelines-February-2024.pdf (accessed February 2024).

UK National Screening Committee (2023). Screening in healthcare. https://www.gov.uk/guidance/principles-of-population-screening/principles-of-screening (accessed January 2024).

UNICEF (2023). Building a happy baby: A guide for parents. The Baby Friendly Initiative & UNICEF. https://www.unicef.org.uk/babyfriendly/baby-friendly-resources/relationship-building-resources/building-a-happy-baby (accessed August 2024).

Welsh Government (2023). Social services activity: April 2021 to March 2022. https://www.gov.wales/sites/default/files/pdf-versions/2023/2/1/1675687678/social-services-activity-april-2021-march-2022.pdf (accessed February 2024).

WHO (2021). WHO calls for better hand hygiene and other infection control practices. World Health Organisation. https://www.who.int/news/item/05-05-2021-who-calls-for-better-hand-hygiene-and-other-infection-control-practices (accessed February 2024).

WHO (2022). WHO launches first ever global report on infection prevention and control. World Health Organisation. https://www.who.int/news/item/06-05-2022-who-launches-first-ever-global-report-on-infection-prevention-and-control (accessed February 2024).

WHO (2024). Head circumference for age. World Health Organisation. https://www.who.int/tools/child-growth-standards/standards/head-circumference-for-age (accessed February 2024).

Yim, S., Petersen, T., Uppal Munawnara Talat and Quinlivan, J. (2023) Compliance of vacuum-assisted delivery. *Australian New Zealand Journal of Obstetric Gynaecology*. 63, pp. 13–18

Ziobro J and Shellhaas RA. (2020) Neonatal seizures: Diagnosis, etiologies, and management. *Seminars in Neurology*, **40** (2): 246–256. https://doi.org/10.1055/s-0040-1702943.

Useful websites

- ICON programme: https://iconcope.org
- The Lullaby Trust – research and information on sudden infant death syndrome: www.lullabytrust.org.uk
- National Bereavement Care Pathway – guidelines: www.teddyswish.org
- National Child Mortality Database: www.ncmd.info
- Personal Child Health Record – information and PCHR images: https://www.healthforallchildren.com/the-pchr and https://www.blmkhealthiertogether.nhs.uk/application/files/6616/1356/1037/167711_v4.5_PCHR_FINAL_complete_Dec_19.pdf
- UK Health Security Agency – routine childhood immunisation schedule: https://www.gov.uk/government/publications/routine-childhood-immunisation-schedule

Useful elearning resources

NHS England's elearning for healthcare (elfh) provides two courses for professionals that are re-evaluated and updated (approx. two-yearly). They can be found via the elfh portal:

https://portal.e-lfh.org.uk/Catalogue/Index?HierarchyId=0_43661_43663&programmeId=43661

The two courses are:

- **Bereavement care after pregnancy loss or baby death – learning for all**. This course provides an introduction to bereavement care and is available for anyone involved in such circumstances.
- **Bereavement care after pregnancy loss or baby death – healthcare professionals**. A follow-on course for healthcare professionals with the aim of raising the standard of knowledge and understanding in relation to providing excellent bereavement care.

There is a newborn blood spot elearning module available when logged into the elfh hub:

https://www.elfh.org.uk/programmes/nhsscreeningprogrammes/#:~:text=The%20NHS%20Newborn%20Blood%20Spot,sickle%20cell%20disease%20(SCD)

Index

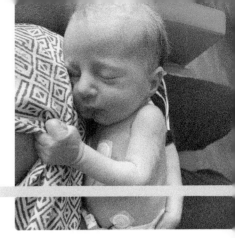

Physical Examination of the Newborn at a Glance, Second Edition. Dr Lyn Dolby and Denise (Dee) Campbell.
© 2025 John Wiley & Sons Ltd. Published 2025 by John Wiley & Sons Ltd.